Back To The Basics

If you're looking for the answer to any (or all) of these questions, and more…..this book is for you.

- How do I stay motivated so I don't fall off the healthy eating wagon?
- How do I stop cravings…especially on the weekends?
- How do I get rid of stubborn belly fat?
- How do I lose fat for good!?
- What is the right portion size for me?
- What should I be feeding my kids?
- Should I or my kids be taking supplements? If so, which ones?
- Are all carbs bad and is sugar toxic?
- Is coffee good or bad for me?
- Am I getting enough protein?
- Can I eat_____________? The answer is in this book.
- Should I be using protein powders? This answer will shock you!
- Do I need to be consuming dairy products?
- Do my kids need cow's milk?
- Should I be tracking macros?
- Should I be doing keto?
- Should I be intermittent fasting?
- Do I need a pre-workout drink?
- Do I need a post-workout drink?
- Most importantly – all the conflicting advice out there is so confusing. Who do I believe??

When you are done with this book all you're going to ask is "Why hasn't anyone made this so easy for me to understand and apply before?"

Dr. Steve Czys

Editing by DocEditing.com

ISBN: 978-0-578-23256-0

This book is presented to

____

by

____

because I care about you and your health

Contents

Preface

I wrote this book because I'm so sick and tired of diet, fitness, and supplement industries spewing out garbage information for profit. People are confused by and then taken advantage of by these companies who sell them foolish diet plans and magic supplements.

Countless people I've worked with have said to me, "I've tried it all, and nothing works!" So, I give them the answers and make them simple to understand and apply. And FINALLY – something works!! The weight comes off, the energy shoots through the roof, confidence soars and all of the confusion disappears.

This book will give you clarity. There will be no more confusion about what to do. I am going, to as it's often said, "teach you how to fish." You will know exactly what foods to buy, how much to eat, what to eat, the best exercise to burn fat, and most importantly, how to hold yourself accountable and never fall of the wagon! Everything you need to achieve the healthy body you've been wanting is in this book. The craziest part is that you will save a bunch of money in the process.

You may be thinking that you've tried everything, and nothing has worked. I can look you straight in the eye and tell you with absolute confidence that NEVER has a person gone all in with my program and told me they didn't see improvement. Not a single one. You won't be the first.

I want you to know I have been there with you. I accepted a great deal of bad advice from so-called "experts." In my twenties, I had terrible digestive issues, asthma, allergies, chronic sinus troubles, almost constant joint pain and snored terribly. I feel far better today in my forties!

I've done all of the hard work figuring out the secret, which I like to call a "cheat code." I feel like I have the cheat code for feeling and looking amazing. It's hard to believe how simple it can be.

You will finish this book overflowing with hope! And you will achieve the look, confidence, and health you've been searching for!

I have one favor to ask: After you apply the simple tools in this book and get amazing results, please tell me about them! Helping others achieve amazing results is what brings me the most joy. You can find me at www.drczys.com. Thank You!

Acknowledgements

Thank you to my amazing wife, Amber. She is great at everything that I am terrible at, which is pretty much everything. Without her, none of this—my book, Eupraxia, my sanity—would be possible. My kids, Zayn and Zary, motivate me every single day. My No. 1 Goal in life is to make them proud of me.

There are so many remarkable people I have learned invaluable lessons from. Most of them have no idea how much of an impact they've had on my life. I was almost ready to quit chiropractic school until I heard Dr. Chestnut speak. Dr. DeMartini, as well, really helped me gain clarity and pursue what I truly wanted to do.

I could fill a chapter just naming the countless other researchers and incredible people that I have learned from. If you are working hard at something, keep grinding. You may have no idea who you are influencing.

Chapter 1: Purpose of This Book

YOU ARE CONSTANTLY BEING LIED TO FOR PROFIT

"Nutrition is really simple, but we insist on making it complicated." – Dr. Steve Czys

Hey, I get it. There's so much conflicting advice all over the internet when it comes to nutrition and exercise. What the hell is a person really supposed to believe? It's maddening, right? Sometimes you get overwhelmed, frustrated, and just want to say, "The heck with it."

I've worked with thousands of people and have heard it countless times, and I understand. Here's what I've done for you: I've read and studied nutrition and exercise, obsessively. This is all I've done for the past two decades. I'm going to take all that confusion, all the nonsense, and I'm going to filter through it and give you the answers. I'm going to make it really simple and easy for you to understand and more importantly, apply.

The purpose of my book is to make it so easy that you almost can't believe it and think, "Oh my God, it can't really be that easy, can it?" Yes, it really can.

People try to confuse you because if you're confused, they can sell you their products. If you're confused and not sure what to do, it's easy to sell you this powder or shake or drink, or that plan, or their NEW gimmick. But, when you have the answer, when someone really teaches you and makes the solution easy, the nonsense immediately sets off your bullshit detector. Now, you think to yourself, "There's no way; that just doesn't make any sense. I'm not going to buy that product."

That's where I'm at and that's where I'm going to take you.

To me, nutrition and exercise are really, really simple. It's become really easy to ignore the noise and the nonsense. And it's become simple to maintain a healthy, fit physique. I'm 41 years old and have the same physique I had when I was 20 because I apply what I'm about to teach you in this book.

"Simplicity is the ultimate sophistication." - Unknown

If you're like me, you like to know the why behind everything. You want to understand things. If you know the why and understand, it's easier to make the right decisions. I must know why I'm doing something, otherwise I won't do it.

On the other hand, you may be different. You may be thinking, "Hey, show me what to do and I'll do it. I don't need to know why. Just give me a step-by-step plan and I'll follow it. I'm ready for the great results." If that's you, just flip to the step-by-step plan at the end of the book. I've laid out a step-by-step, easy-to-follow plan for you.

So, you have two options. You can start here and gain the understanding behind diet, nutrition and exercise (which I recommend). I make it really simple, so you truly understand the secrets to healthy living. Or, you can just skip to the end and apply the **cheat code.** I've laid it out for you. Exactly what groceries to go buy, exactly what meals to make. I show you exactly how to do it in the most cost-effective way, because eating healthy doesn't have to be crazy expensive.

If you just follow the plan, in 6 weeks you're going to drop at least 20 pounds if you have 20 pounds to lose. I guarantee it. You may be thinking, "Oh that's crazy, I've tried everything." You haven't tried this! I have helped countless people reach their goals. Throughout this book, you will meet a number of people, just like you, who are now at their ideal body size and have completely different lives even though previously, nothing worked for them.

Remember playing video games and entering a cheat code that gave your character super powers that made the game easier to play or beat? That's what this book is. It's the **cheat code** to feeling amazing! I've done all the work and made it easy for you!

It's Not Your Fault

You are going to learn things in this book that will shock you. You may feel guilty about some of the foods you have been eating and/or feeding your kids. I want to make sure that you know it's not your fault! You have been lied to and have been doing what you thought was best. Big businesses and very clever marketers are very good at spreading lies. I have been duped as well. I can't believe some of the foolish things I've paid for in the past.

The good news is that it won't happen again. Once you've read this book, you'll have the knowledge to reveal the BS that big business is trying to sell you!

THE A-HA! MOMENT THAT CHANGED MY LIFE

"The ultimate in sophistication is simplicity." - Leonard Thiessen

How did I get here? I'm going to tell you a little story. Throughout my practice as a chiropractor, I realized that what just about all of my patients really needed wasn't another prescription or adjustment or X-ray, but instead, what I've been doing for myself. A healthy diet, better exercise, and a more grateful attitude was the answer. Proper nutrition and exercise were what just about everybody was missing. Patients' joints hurt, they experienced headaches, their energy was low, their sex drive was low, they were overweight, they didn't feel good, and were sick and tired of being sick and tired! All of these issues really came down to two important factors: exercise and good nutrition.

The big turning point for me happened when I was at a conference for doctors in Chicago. It was supposed to be a health conference, but most doctor's conferences I've been to are usually all about marketing and billing insurance to maximize income, and it's freaking maddening.

As I was looking around the room, it became very apparent that very few doctors were actually healthy. They were overweight, drinking sodas and eating bagels, and very few looked vibrant and healthy. How was it that health providers couldn't stay healthy? That was crazy. Think about it. Would you ever ask a broke financial advisor for financial advice? I would hope not. That would be insane. Would you take your car to an auto mechanic who drives a hoopty of a car in constantly poor condition? I would hope not. Would you go to a dentist who has bad teeth? Yet, people commonly seek nutrition and health advice from unhealthy and overweight healthcare providers. It's insane.

What made the healthy doctors in that room healthy? Proper diet and exercise! They ate right and exercised. So, I told myself, "When I get home, I'm going to open a whole new facility using a program that will be laser-focused on teaching people how to eat the right way, how to exercise, and as simple and easy to apply as possible." And I did just that by opening Eupraxia. Very quickly, we grew to seven locations, and continue to grow. The reason is because the results people in this program are achieving are hard to believe. Anyone who applies what's in this book, what I teach, will get amazing results. Not once has a person told me they applied what I taught them and didn't feel better. *Not once!*

I just want you to know I'm nothing special, not one bit. I'm truly no different than you are. I gain weight really easy. You know those people who can gain weight just by looking at a cookie? I'm one of those people. I have injuries like you. I've had multiple knee surgeries, hip surgery, and shoulder surgery, following a few of my many sport injuries.

I have low points and lapses in motivation just like you. Sometimes I just don't feel like doing anything. Sometimes I allow myself to care what others think of me. I too worry about being judged.

I have two kids and know how crazy busy it can get with kids, work, a broken car, a washed-out driveway, and the many problems of life we all face. If I can do it, so can you. I'm no different than you and definitely nothing special. I have no superior gifts or powers and I'm definitely not a better person than you. The secret is that through it all, I will still take action, and I will show you the exact actions I take to get results that I also want you to get. You can absolutely get the exact same results I do.

What's really amazing is when people come to me for weight loss and their rheumatoid arthritis disappears; or their eczema disappears; their plantar fasciitis disappears, their shoulder pain disappears, their irritable bowel syndrome, Crohn's disease, fibromyalgia, depression and anxiety disappears. It's astonishing. A lot of people have told me about how their brain fog just went away completely. So many people have started this program for weight loss, yet it's their other health problems that have improved so much; the weight loss was just a bonus. With this plan, it's not what you lose but what you gain that really matters.

Here's what's beautiful about what I teach and what's in this book: The way you should be eating is the same way your husband, your wife, your kids, or your grandkids should be eating. The same foods, just different portions.

The big difference between this book and other weight loss books out there is that in this book, I ask the RIGHT question: What is the healthiest diet for humans?

The WRONG question asks what you should eat to lose weight. That's why there are so many crazy diet plans available. They all ask the wrong question. That's also why so many of them are terribly unhealthy and lead to gaining even more weight shortly after trying them.

When you eat for your health, you become healthier, you look better, you feel better and weight loss is an amazing side effect.

This is the way I eat. This is also the way my wife and toddler eat. This is also the way our baby's going to eat once she gets off mom's boob. In fact, she's eating like us now because she's eating the food that mom eats through breastfeeding. So, all four of us are eating the exact same foods, only in different portions. I will go into detail about portion sizes for you. On average, American portions are enormous. Often, a "small" meal is actually quite large.

If you want to stop here and go buy groceries for your week-one plan now, go ahead! Let's get you snacking on the best foods while you read the rest!

But, why the hell should you believe anything I have to say? Because this is all I've ever done. I still have workouts I wrote when I was 14 years old. I maxed out attending school, earned my doctorate, have been in practice as a chiropractor for many years, have spent decades obsessing about and studying nutrition, exercise and mindset, and MOST IMPORTANTLY helping tons of people just like you achieve great results.

I feel it is very important that I practice what I preach. The old adage says, "A pint of example is worth a gallon of advice." Everything that I teach, I do, to a tee. I think this is vital because there are a lot of frauds out there. They're taking steroids and telling you to take this magic pill or that supplement, or this shake. They're cheating and trying to sell you something else. What I teach is exactly what I do. If you come into my home at any minute of any day, you would find in my cupboards, fridge, and meals exactly the foods you're about to read about. These photos show me at 30 and at 40.

I'm going to let you in on a little secret: Fit does not equal healthy! When I was a young buck, I played loads of sports and trained like a madman. My physique was great...but I was sick. Allergies, asthma, chronic digestive issues, chronic sinus issues, joint pain, snoring; I was clueless when it came to eating for health.

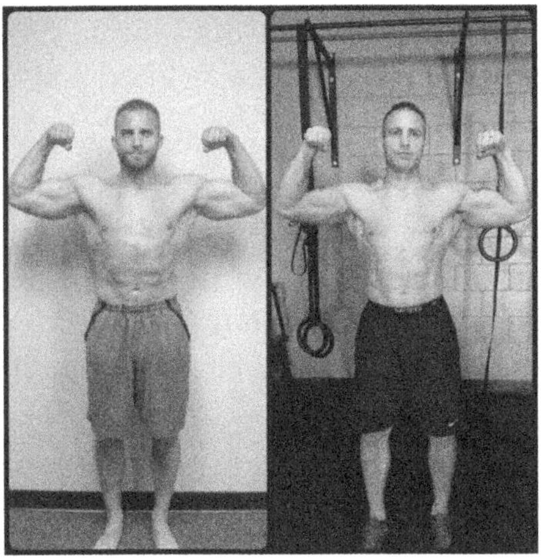

It's possible to be fit on a bad diet but you cannot be HEALTHY on a bad diet! I suffered through a lot of pain before figuring out that what I eat is far more important than how much I eat. I now feel better at 40 than I did at 20!

THEY TRIED EVERYTHING AND FAILED, UNTIL THIS

Meet Roger

Roger is 67 years old. I want you to visualize how awesome his day is: First, you get a workout in. Then you either go golfing, hiking, or hang out with your grandkids all day. Your grandkids are toddlers and they call you "active grandpa" because you do so much fun stuff with them. Then you go on a 50-mile bike ride because you can, and you enjoy it. Nod your head up and down if this would be awesome. YES! An amazing retirement.

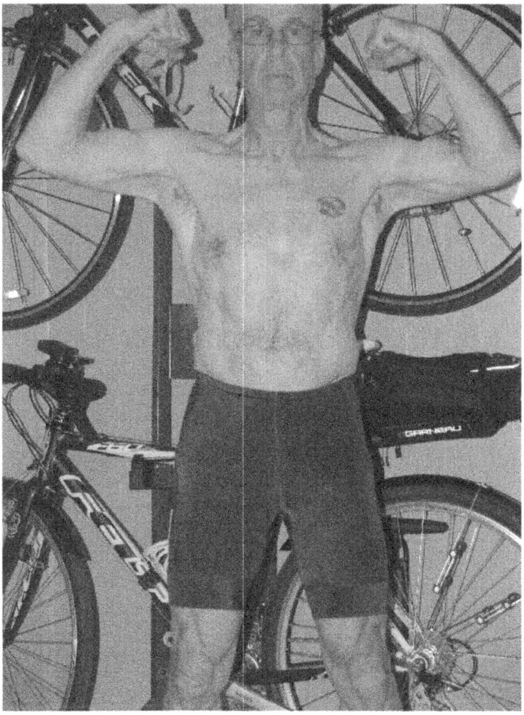

How many people at 67 are barely moving and spending most of their week going to doctor appointments? I say, to heck with that! Make the right choices now to make your future amazing!

Here's a crazy statistic for you to think about. The life expectancy in the US is about 77 years old. Over the last two years, it has actually dropped! For the first time in history, our kids are not expected to live as long as their parents! It gets worse.

What about the "functional" life expectancy in the US? On average, at what age are Americans no longer able to take care of themselves? **64!** That's not living in my opinion. It doesn't have to be that way. Make the right choices and your life can be like Roger's.

Crazy Fact: On average, two people die, and four babies are born every second.

His life is more active and more enjoyable than many 20-year-olds' lives. All of us have that potential and that motivates the shit out of me! What do I want retirement to be like? Sitting around in a chair watching TV? Or LIVING! Playing with my grandkids, loving the shit out of life! I will explain to you how genetics plays a very tiny role in what your future looks like. YOU have the POWER to dictate your future quality of life. I'm going to show you how what you eat can change your genetic expression and exactly *what* to eat to maximize your genetic potential. How great does that sound?

It gets even better: the process to achieve that is enjoyable! And the years leading up to retirement are also more enjoyable.

Karen's Story

"Looking back on my first year with Dr. Czys, one memory in particular comes to mind. Running, jumping and sliding in the park with my four-year-old grandson. The freedom of being able to follow him and play, seeing the joy in his eyes as his 'Gammy' copies his every move! Then I flash back to the moment I decided to join Dr. Czys and Eupraxia. I woke up sick, tired and bloated. I didn't want to feel that way anymore or ever again. I couldn't sleep, had constant heartburn, even with medication, and uncontrolled asthma.

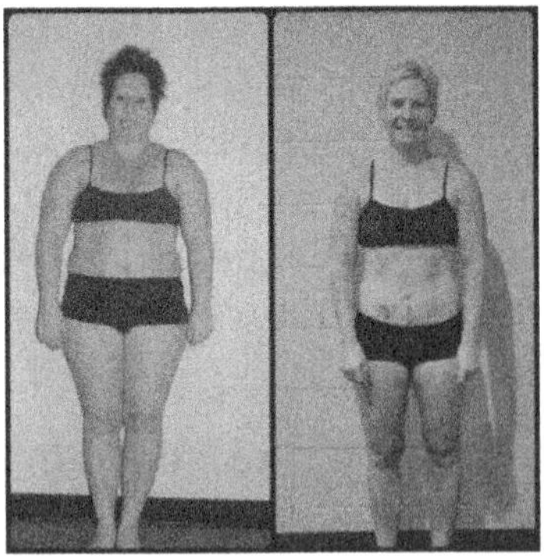

"One year, 66 pounds and 18 inches off my waist later, I no longer require medication to sleep or for my heartburn, my asthma is practically nonexistent, and I feel amazing! Dr. Czys' lectures include a segment about finding a purpose, a reason to improve and focusing on it. If I could say one thing to a person just starting out, be patient, keep your eye on your purpose and fulfill it! Change will come slow at first perhaps, but then like a stroll (or run) in the park, it will get easier!"

Will

I want you to look at Will's face. This was after just four months in my program and look how much younger he looks. What I teach in this book is the fountain of youth. Instead of buying all of the antiaging creams and potions and lotions out there, if you want to look younger and feel younger, follow this program. Just look at Will's face. He took ten years off in just four months. It's absolutely amazing. What was really cool was that Will had blood work done before and after following the eating plan. After, his cholesterol was down 50 points and his triglycerides were down 100. Weight was down, and blood pressure was down. All of this happened just by following what's in this book.

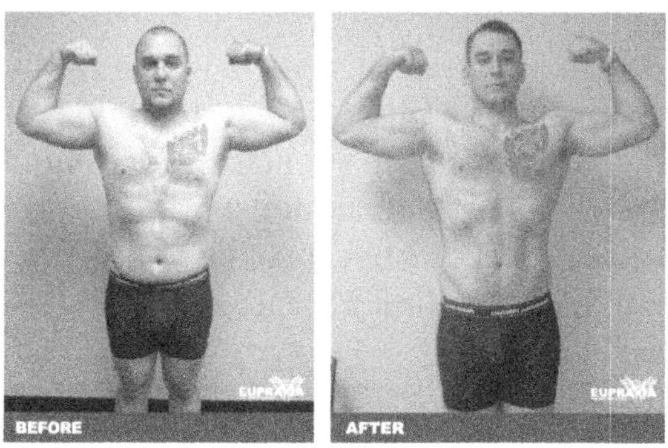

Will isn't an anomaly, either. Check out Bryan who also looks a decade younger.

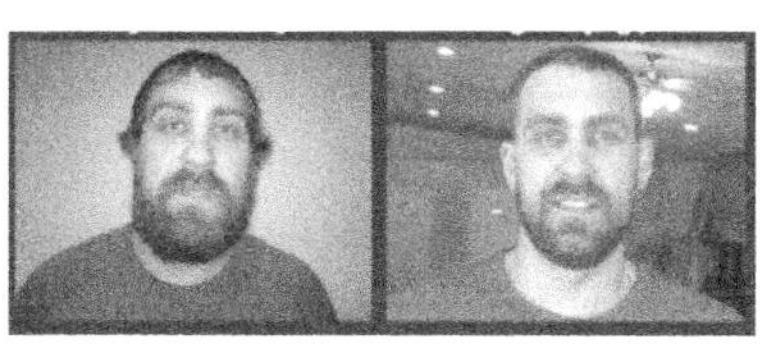

Darci

This lovely woman is a mother of five.

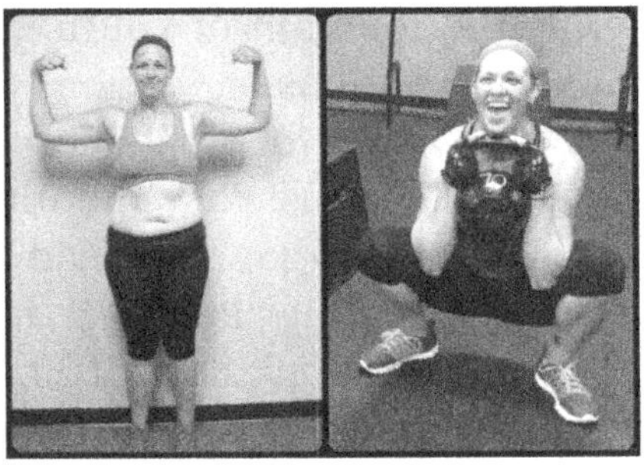

I always love to share this picture for two reasons. One, Darci looks freaking amazing and often I hear the line, "Oh, but I have kids." Perfect! I see no greater REASON to become healthier than because you have kids! I guarantee you that the better choices you make will trickle down to the little ones and make their lives much better too.

Another reason I love showing this pic is to point out the big weight she's holding onto. One of the things ladies don't do nearly enough of is weight training. Typically, women spend countless hours on the cardio machine hamster wheel—the absolute worst way to burn fat—and then avoid lifting heavy weights because they think it will give them big muscles. Here's the truth; and I'll get into details later. Lifting weights is the BEST way to burn fat!!

Lindsey

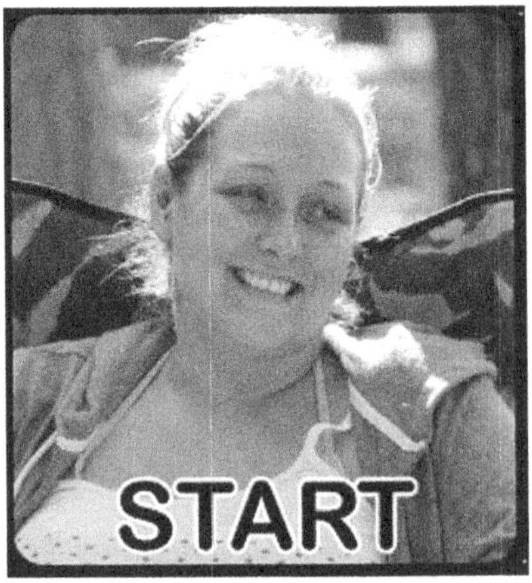

Next, is my right-hand woman, Lindsey. This is a really inspiring story I love sharing. Lindsey came to my clinic because of a car accident. She had neck pain from whiplash. She came to me for neck pain but my goal for everyone isn't just to relieve their pain. It's to get them healthy! So, we sat down and talked like all health care providers should do with their patients.

I discovered she was on anxiety medications and anti-depressants, following the food pyramid, jogging all the time and doing all the things she thought were needed to lose weight. She was eating lots of whole grains and watching her fat intake.

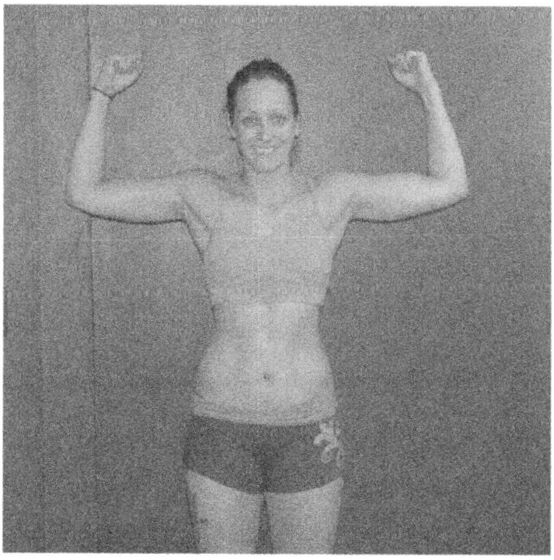

The problem was that it wasn't working, and she felt like crap. So, I showed her how to do it the right way and look at her six months later. And she's maintained it four years later. She's been working with me for years. The change in her life is amazing. She did it by following the plan in the book. The real secret is that she *applied* it! Check out this young lady now; pretty awesome change, right? Now she's a fitness trainer!

Keith

Now, this next story is extremely important. When Keith first started, he could barely lift his one arm above his head. His shoulder had been severely damaged in an accident. He started off with very basic exercises and slowly but surely kept getting stronger and stronger. Before he knew it, the guy was knocking out push-ups and doing pull-ups in his sixties.

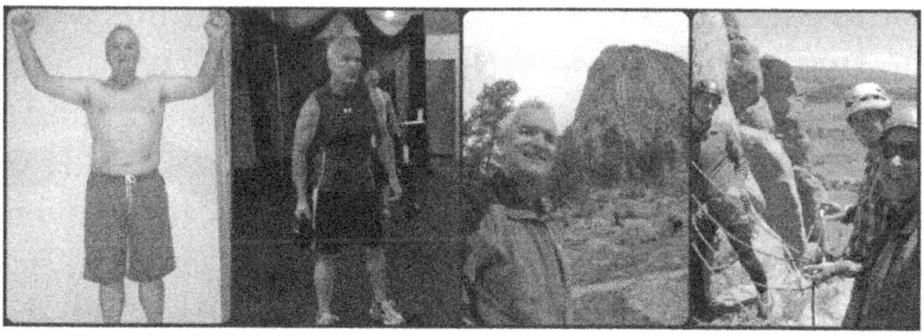

Check out what he's doing now. Here's Keith climbing cliff faces with his sons in Utah. Talk about an amazing transformation in quality of life. Imagine going from barely lifting your arm to travelling west and climbing mountains with your sons! That's what this plan is really all about, and what you'll be able to do because of your body changes that matters. You'll get to experience so much more in life.

Mark

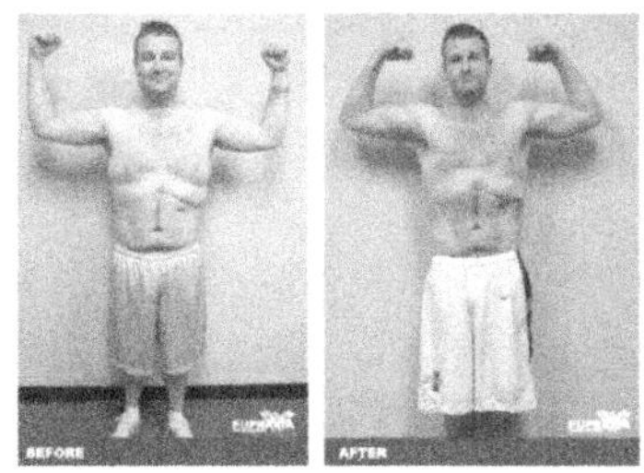

This next story is scary! When I met Mark, I was speaking at a presentation in Madison, WI. He just happened to sit next to me, and we started chatting. In his early thirties, Mark had a heart attack. That was his wake-up call. "Holy shit, I need to do something different."

Here's the deal. I don't want you to wait until tragedy happens to make changes. Do it right now! Not this weekend or next month. Now! Too many people wait until they experience a tragedy before they make a change, and for him it was almost too late. Often, people don't get a second chance. Don't wait. Just apply it now. The timing is never perfect, there is always other stuff going on. You just have to apply it now.

Donna

This is what 110 pounds down looks like. Do you think she feels much, much better? She just followed the program. The biggest thing for Donna was the eating. Note: She "only" lost two pounds a week. That's it. Just about two pounds a week. Nice and steady. Two pounds a week

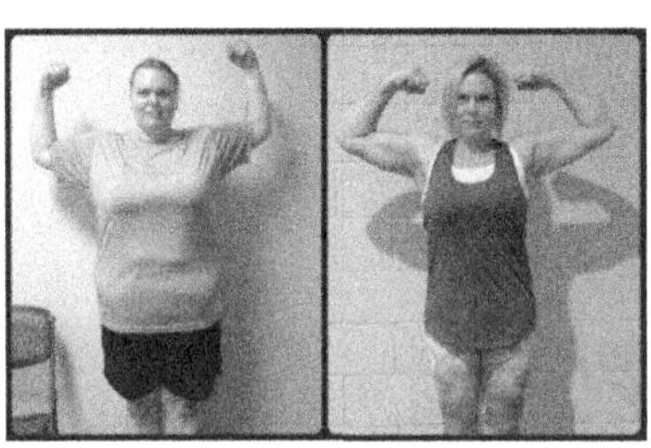

times 52 weeks in a year and that's 104 pounds. That's how quickly you can be down 100 pounds. It can even be faster than that. Too often, people get discouraged, saying, "Oh, I only lost two pounds a week." Only?! Stick with it for a year and boom, down 104.

Ben

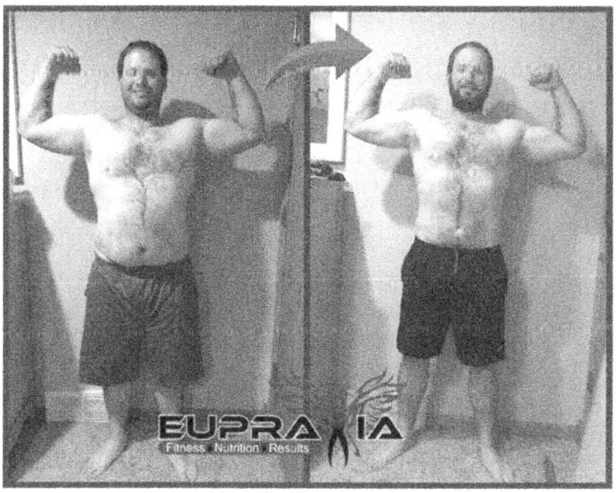

"Back in January of last year (2018) I went on a dream vacation. My wife and I were over in London and we were miserable. We were walking everywhere and were getting tired and it was just the second day of ten. That is where it started, and I realized that I needed to do something.

"One day at work it was even worse, and I thought to myself that I needed to do something now. I was also having chronic back pain at about the same time and found out that I had two compressed discs in my back. I had a buddy that had just finished up a six-week challenge and he felt and looked great. He had been giving me a hard time and I finally asked him what it was all about. At first, I was a little leery. But I knew I needed to do something and Eupraxia fit what I was looking for. They showed me how to eat healthy and had a great environment.

"I finally took the step and started my challenge April 21, 2018 and have never looked back. I have gotten rid of 60 pounds and feel great. I raced in a 10K and a Spartan: two things that I never thought I would do. And this year I am going to complete a Spartan Trifecta! Thanks, you guys have given me time back with my boys."

Joe

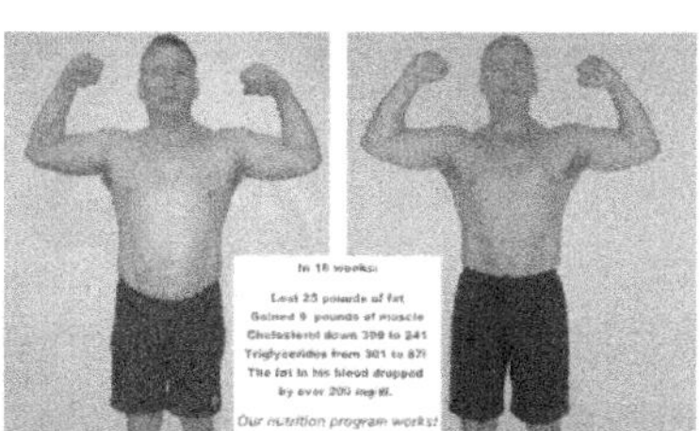

Joe, 52-years old; looks great, right? Obviously, his body change is awesome. But what's really crazy is that his cholesterol went down 70 points and his triglycerides, the fat in his blood, dropped over 200 points. Those are life-extending, lifesaving changes!

Malissa

Let's learn from Malissa. You're reading the book, and you're excited, you're pumped, and can't wait to get started. That's great—you should be because this is going to change your life! When Malissa began, she lost some weight. Then she gained a little bit back and then she lost some again and then she gained some back. So, she was on that rollercoaster many people end up on. Finally, she decided, "You know what? I'm just going to start being CONSISTENT with everything."

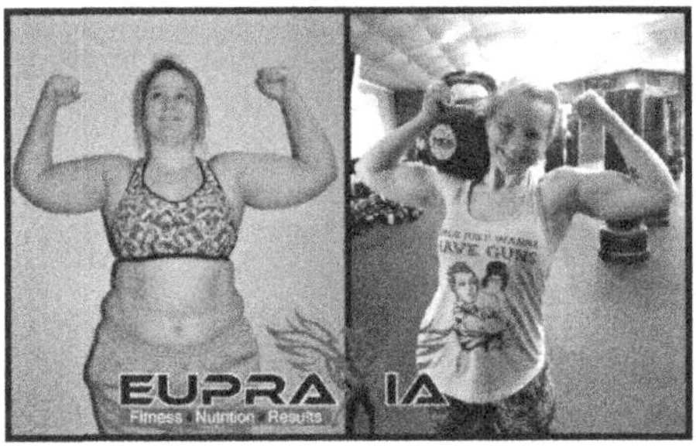

And look what happened. That's how you find the magic. You need to realize this picture shows what going all in consistently—NOT half-assed—will do. Massive, massive changes.

Marianne

Often, I hear, "God, I wish I could have my 20-year-old body back." You can. Just do what's laid out in the book! Check out this 20-year-old body...on a 38-year-old mom! She had some kids and let herself go a bit. Then Marianne decided to get serious and start eating healthy, as taught in this book. Boom. Look at that body—amazing. Exactly the same as she was back in college, minus the tan. Pretty awesome results.

"We were a busy family with four young boys. I ran a business from home, served on two local boards of directors and volunteered at a local non-profit. I was exhausted, but my husband convinced me it was something we could do together. If I was honest with myself, I would admit that at that point in my life, it had been years since I had felt good at all. I had recently been diagnosed with an autoimmune condition that left me feeling continually tired; I had no mental clarity and struggled with fogginess and poor memory. I had gained significant weight, I had eczema on my abdomen and my adult acne was the worst it had ever been. I was struggling with depression. Every fall I would be plagued with bronchitis that would last for six to eight weeks and would take several prescription antibiotics to finally clear. At just 36 years old, I was beginning to realize that if I didn't address my health, I wasn't going to live the life I desired. I was ready for change, and Eupraxia would find me at just the right time.

"It finally clicked. I remember sitting in on the nutrition talk with Dr. Czys and listening to his evidence on the problems with sugar, grains and dairy. I started going through my favorite family recipes in my head and substituting yellow potatoes with sweet potatoes, pasta with zucchini noodles, and ditching the side of bread. My roasted chicken with vegetables, favorite kale soup, and best meatloaf could all be tweaked to work. I felt the mental shift...I COULD DO THIS! Unlike every other diet I had tried, which focused on deprivation (low fat, low calorie), I could enjoy healthy fats, fruits, vegetables, and meat and eat when I felt hungry. My husband and I would start that day. We would begin just cutting out sugar and grains, because I needed a "Keep it simple stupid" approach. The first 10 days were the hardest, but soon new habits were forming, and it would become more like second nature. I would eventually cut out dairy a few months later.

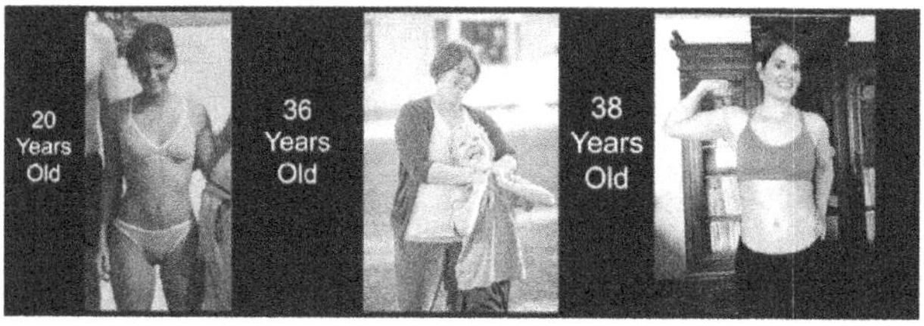

"Things started happening. Within the first month of sticking to the new dietary changes and working out 3-5 days a week at Eupraxia, I would lose 6 pounds of body fat and 6 inches off my waist. I started supplementing with the fish oil, vitamin D and the quality probiotics offered by Dr. Czys to optimize my health. Within five months, I would be down more than 20 pounds in body fat, had lowered my cholesterol from 236 to 205, my energy increased, my sleep improved, my mental clarity improved, and my depression started to lift. Over a year into this life change now, I am down 38 pounds of body fat, I am stronger, doing full floor pushups and conquering those box jumps. Every single one of my health struggles has been dramatically improved, if not eliminated by changing how I eat and move.

"Looking to the future: The ability to improve my health and well being through food and exercise has felt immensely empowering. I feel free; no longer a slave to my old health and my old body, or some uncontrollable situation. I could grab the bull by the horns, put in the hard work with consistency and effort and change my life. I was in control. Looking to the future, I feel hopeful about what the next 36 years will look like. It's the kind of thing that starts to impact every other area of your life. I am still amazed by it, and grateful for it every single day."

Kim

I'd like you to meet Kim. This is her Facebook profile picture. In the photo on the right, she is obviously proud of finishing a Spartan race.

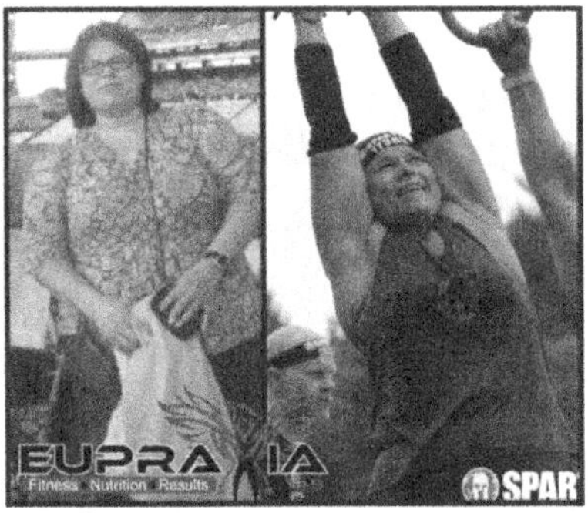

When she started with me, she weighed over 300 pounds. Her original picture shows that she couldn't have made it up the first hill of the Spartan Race. After my program, she completed the whole damn race and almost all the obstacles. She was so happy and felt so good afterwards. "I can't wait to do the next one," was the first thing she said. That's what life is all about. That's why these changes are so, so important.

Lian

"My journey with health has not been a straight path; in fact for some reason, I think I've chosen most of my life to make things the MOST difficult for myself. In high school, I was 100% in the mindset of being better than everyone else, no matter the cost on my body. Especially regardless of the cost on my overall heath. The thick-skulled mindset I had then played incredibly into my poor decisions in college.

"College was a slap in the face for me, and after years of doing meal replacement shakes, the Keto diet, counting my macros, literally everything and anything I read on the internet that PROMISED and swore with a money back guarantee to either improve my digestive issues and weight problems ultimately failed me completely. I didn't try to get the hundreds and hundreds of dollars back that I'd spent on those products, but instead I gave up. I quit working out, quit eating healthy, and quit eating at all sometimes, unfortunately.

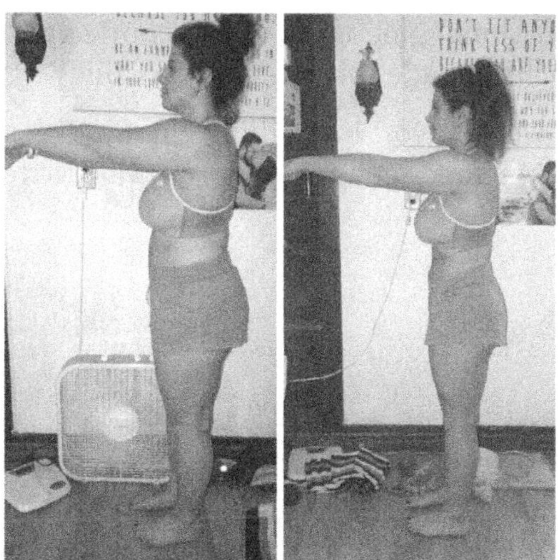

"When I came across Dr. Czys on Facebook and saw the results people were getting, I really wanted to figure out how to make that exact progress for myself. I tell myself and others that I just did it—I started with the six-week challenge not even realizing that I was about to completely change my life!"

"After three weeks into the challenge, I noticed that not just a *few* of my symptoms of diagnosed Crohn's disease were gone, but ALL of my symptoms were gone!!

"The chronic disease I was in the hospital for at the start of the year had since seemed to heal completely only three weeks after I'd begun eating the way Dr. Czys taught and working my ass off in the workouts. By the end of my six weeks, I was off of my infusions (done dealing with the hassle of the bills for those infusions, $2,500 every 3 weeks) and I finally realized why I challenged myself. And finally—I found my happiness. Now almost 40 pounds down, I can't imagine my life any other way. Food truly is meant to heal, not harm your body. I don't know where I would be right now without Dr. Czys' constant guidance and support. I'm so happy to have found my happy place."

Shelly

"I joined with intentions of just successfully completing the six-week challenge. The nutritional guidance (which is priceless!) and the meal plans with grocery lists made it very simple to follow.

"Within the first week or two, I had a different mindset on commitment as I was already seeing and feeling changes. I was excited to go to class each time."

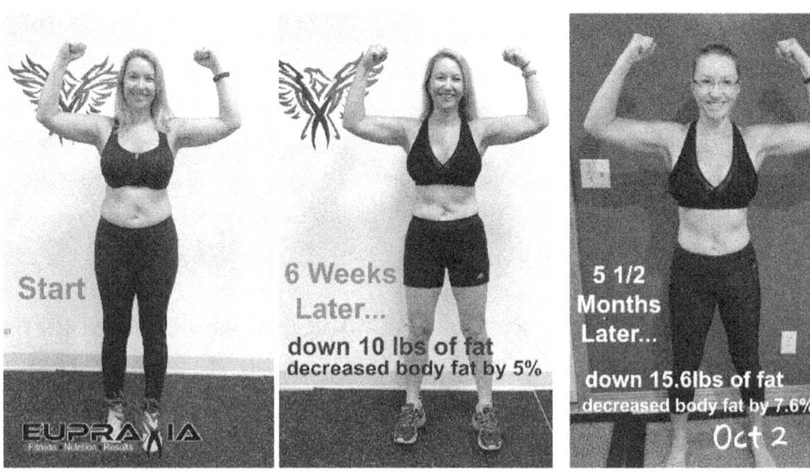
Start
6 Weeks Later...
down 10 lbs of fat
decreased body fat by 5%
5 1/2 Months Later...
down 15.6lbs of fat
decreased body fat by 7.6%
Oct 2

"My Crohn's disease symptoms were minimized! And I no longer have blood sugar issues which is due to the change of diet.

"I gained confidence in myself as I dropped body fat and even gained muscle. My family has also benefited as we eat healthier and have the nutritional education to make better choices.

"There are no gimmicks or quick fixes to good health. You get authentic advice with a great support system during and following the challenge. The trainers and gym peeps at Eupraxia are uplifting and supportive which makes it's very easy to walk through the door each time."

Where Can I Find True Happiness?

I could go on and on and on, sharing examples. If you'd like to read about more of them, visit eupraxia.us/success-stories. Reading about the success of others, especially people who were in the same situation as you are now, is motivating. "If they can do it, I can do it!"

It's not about what you lose – It's about what you gain!

Why lose the weight? What is it really about? Isn't the purpose to have a much higher quality of life? To truly be happy with ourselves inside and out?

Where does happiness come from? True happiness comes from experiences and especially from experiences with the people we care about. The more you experience with others, the happier you will be. Science has proven this time and time again.

Happiness is not about having more stuff. Retail therapy has never and will never make anyone happy long term. We are constantly being sold on retail therapy: If we just buy more stuff, we'll be happier. But this theory just doesn't work. The best investment you can make is in yourself. Not in the amount of stuff you pile up.

Marketers also expect us to believe that simply by having more money, we'll be happier. Studies have shown that once a family's income reaches $70,000 per year, any amount earned over that doesn't improve happiness. A family that brings in 70 million is no happier than a family bringing in $70,000!

When you are fit and healthy, you have the chance to experience more, much more! And when you can do more, your kids can do more. Countless women have told me how awesome it was that they could now play WITH their kids, as opposed to only watching them play. They can now go on the hikes they used to avoid. They can go to the waterpark without being self-conscious. They are DOING instead of sitting back and watching!

Chapter 2: You Will Not Read a More Important Chapter

The Most Important First Step That Every Other Diet Plan Is Missing

Have you ever tried a diet or fitness program to get healthier and then quit later? Nod your head up and down if it's a yes. Are you nodding with me? Have you fallen off the wagon a few times? Yes? Nod your head up and down. Guess what: you're not alone. Every single person I've worked with has as well. So, the question is how do we keep from falling off the wagon? What is the best strategy to stay motivated and to stick with the plan? Seriously, what's the point of starting if you're just going to stop and end up right back where you started? What good is all the great information in this book if it's not applied?

Remember that old adage, "Knowledge is power"? It's not true. Knowledge plus **action** is power. If you have knowledge, yet you don't put it into action it's useless. It serves no purpose. So, how do you act on the knowledge and maintain the action? How do you stay on the wagon? Finding your "Why" is, by far, the best way to do exactly that.

I want you to think about what you care about the most. What do you think about the most often? What are most of the pictures around your house, on your phone, that you share on Facebook of? What do you like to talk about the most? What do you spend the most money on? Where do you spend most of your time? If you have kids, the answer is definitely your kids. But there is no wrong answer. Maybe it's your career. Maybe it's your spouse, your nephew, or your grandkids. There's no wrong answer.

For me, it's my kids, so I'm going to use kids as an example. If you have kids, are they the most important thing in your life? Yes? Nod your head up and down. Yes, absolutely. One hundred percent the most important thing in your life. Let me ask you this, would you do anything for your kids? Do you want your kids to be healthy? Yes, of course. Here's what I want you to do.

I want you to first put a picture of your kids on the table in front of you. I then want you to write down 50 ways in which your losing weight, moving better, eating better, feeling better and having more energy will make their lives better. Fifty ways. You must come up with 50 ways and you must write it down by hand. You can't type it. Write down 50 ways in which your application of what's in this book and becoming healthier makes your kids' lives better. This is the secret. Once you attach your improved health to improving whatever you care about the most, you'll never stop. For me, attaching it to what I care about the most is really easy, and that's my kids.

It wasn't always my kids. For a long time, I was driven to excel at sports. Sports kept me motivated for decades until I stopped participating in sports as often. Then my career was my motivator. I knew that if I ate well, got proper sleep, and worked out, I'd have more energy, think clearer, get more done, and advance faster in my career. Now it's all about my family and being the best dad possible.

I know that if I eat healthy, exercise, and take care of myself and if I have more energy, my family members' lives will be better because of it. I also know if I'm tired and overweight and can't get up to play with my kids they will suffer. I know that if I'm eating bad food, they'll be eating bad food. If I'm just sitting around watching TV, they'll be sitting around watching TV. The choices I make have a huge impact on the quality of life of my family. Because of this, you can be damn sure I'll be making the right choices.

That knowledge is so motivating that it makes it easy for me to make healthy choices. One, I'm making their lives better because I can play and do more activities. Two, they're watching me. **Kids may not do what you say but they'll never fail to imitate you.** The best gift you can give your child is to live an active lifestyle. If I'm living an active lifestyle and eating healthy foods, then they're eating healthy foods with me. Does that make their lives better? Yes.

If your kids are living a healthier lifestyle because they're following in your footsteps, will their lives be better? One hundred percent; there is no question about it. You don't want them to ever have weight issues. You don't want them to ever have confidence or self-esteem issues. You want them to be confident, fit, healthy, successful, and happy people. And the way to do this is through leading by example. Once that idea is deep in your subconscious, you will never stop because you just care too damn much.

If you don't have kids, the same principle still applies. What's the most important thing in your life? Is it your work? Is it your pets? Is it your spouse? Is it a cause that you strongly believe in? It doesn't matter what it is. What makes humans beautiful is that we value different things. That's why so many amazing different things are accomplished.

Determining Your Values: A Step-by-Step Guide

If you aren't sure what your highest values are, this exercise will help you find them. Give two or three answers for each question. If you find yourself providing the same answer every time, that's great! You're finding your values! I learned this exercise from Dr. John DeMartini, a smarter man than I'll ever be.

Step One: Answer the following 13 questions

1. How do you fill your personal space?

Have you ever noticed how things that are really not important to you end up in the trash, the attic, or the storage closet? By contrast, you keep the things that are important to you where you can see them, whether at home or at work.

When you look around your home or office, do you see family photos, sports trophies, business awards, or books? Do you see beautiful objects, comfortable furniture for friends to sit on, or souvenirs of your favorite forms of entertainment? Do you see souvenirs from travels? Whatever you see around you are very strong clues to what you value most.

____

____

____

2. How do you spend your time?

People always make time for things that are really important to them and run out of time for things that aren't. Even though people frequently say, "I don't have time for what I really want to do," the truth is that they are too busy doing what is truly most important to them. And what they think they want to be doing isn't usually what's most important. You will always find time for things that are really important to you. Somehow, you figure out how to make it happen.

How do you spend your time? I spend my days playing with my kids, researching fitness and nutrition, or enjoying time in the woods. Those are my three favorite ways to spend time. I always find time for them and I almost never find time for cleaning, shopping, and domestic activities, which are low on my list. How do you like to spend your time?

____

____

____

3. How do you spend your energy?

You always have energy for things that inspire you, the things you value most. You run out of energy quickly for things that you don't value. Things that are low among your values drain you; things that are high among your values energize you. In fact, when you do something that you value highly, you have more energy at the end of the day than when you started because you were doing something that you love and are inspired by. So, how do you spend your energy and what gives you energy?

____

____

____

4. How do you spend your money?

Again, you always find money for things that are valuable to you but resist parting with money for things that are not important to you. Your choices about spending money reveal a great deal about what you value the most. Now, at this point, you might be noticing some overlap and similarities between what you fill your space with and how you spend your time, energy, and money. That is healthy. It means that you have already aligned a lot of your values, goals, and daily activities.

____

____

____

5. Where do you maintain the most order and organization?

We tend to bring order and organization to things that are important to us and to allow chaos and disorder to exist with things that are low on our list of values. Look at where the greatest order and organization can be found in your life, and you'll gain a good sense of what matters to you most. In my case, I see the most order and organization with my hunting and Eupraxia business and in my scheduled workouts. This helps me realize that my values involve health, outdoors, Eupraxia and my kids (everything about the kids is messy ☺).

____

____

____

6. For what parts of your life are you most reliable, disciplined, and focused?

We never need to be reminded by others to do the things that we value the most. We are inspired from within to do those things, and then do them. Examine the activities, relationships, and goals for which you are disciplined, reliable, and focused: things that nobody has to remind or require you to do. For me, yet again, that includes my kids, hunting, working out, and talking about health. I love those things!

7. What do you think about, and what is your most dominant thought?

I'm not talking about the negative self-thought or the things that distract you. I'm not talking about the fantasies, "shoulds," or "oughts." I'm talking about your most common thoughts about how you want your life to be—thoughts that you've shown slow or steady evidence of bringing to fruition.

8. What are you drawn to on social media or the internet?

Again, I'm not talking about fantasies. I'm asking about what you visualize for your life that is slowly but surely coming true. In my case, I visualized speaking in front of crowds and helping thousands of people, my wife and kids, as well as living on and owning a huge farm. And that is also what I am realizing. So, what are you visualizing and realizing?

9. What would you do with a free week and unlimited money?

For me this is easy. I would spend that time and money with my family. How would you spend that time and money? There is no wrong answer!

10. What do you talk about in social settings?

Okay, now here's a way to zero in on your values as you've probably done with other people as well.

What topics do you persistently want to bring into conversation, topics that you don't need any persuasion to talk about? What subjects turn you into an instant extrovert?

You've probably noticed that there are certain topics that immediately bring you to life and get you to start talking, while certain *other* topics turn you into an introvert who has nothing to say or tries to change the subject. You can use this same insight to analyze other people's values. If you approach someone and they ask you about your kids, that means their kids are important to them. If they ask, "How's business?", they value business. If they ask, "Are you seeing anyone new?", then relationships matter to them. Topics that attract you are a key to what you value. This is why I struggle in most group settings. Frequently, the things people like to talk about in groups don't interest me.

____

____

____

11. What inspires you?

What inspires you now? What has inspired you in the past? What is common about the people who inspire you? Figuring out what inspires you the most reveals what you value the most.

____

____

____

12. What are the most consistent long-term goals that you've set?

What two or three long-term goals have you focused on that are becoming a reality? Again, I'm not talking about the fantasies that are not reflected in your life at all. I want to know the dreams you are bringing into reality slowly but surely, the dreams that have been dominating your mind and your thoughts for a while. The dreams that are becoming a part of your daily life, step by step by step.

____

____

____

13. What do you love to learn and read about most?

What three topics do you most often love learning or reading about? What three topics can you stay focused on and love learning about without getting distracted? For example, next to my bed is a stack of books on health, fitness, nutrition, and hunting.

____

____

____

Step Two: Identify the Answers that Have Been Repeated the Most

Once you've provided 2 or 3 answers for each of the 13 questions, you'll notice that among your answers, there is some repetition, perhaps even a great amount of repetition. You may have expressed the same kinds of values in different ways. For example, answers such as "Spending time with people I like", "Having a drink with the folks from work", and "Going out to eat with my friends" appear distinct, but if you look closely, common patterns will emerge.

Find the answer that was repeated most often and beside it, write how many times it was repeated. Then find the second most frequent answer, then the third, and so on, until you have ranked every single answer. This gives you an excellent primary indicator of what your highest values are. You may even start making decisions based on this initial hierarchy of values and discover how your life has already begun demonstrating your commitment to these values.

Your Why and Your Motivation

What is YOUR Why? What is YOUR reason for making a change? What is most important to you?

____

____

Step Three: Determine How this Plan Will Affect Your Life

No matter what or who is the most important thing to you—write down at least 50 ways in which eating better, living healthier, having more energy, and having more confidence benefits whatever you value the most.

How can exercise help what you value the most?

1. ____________________ 2. ____________________

3. ____________________ 4. ____________________

5. ____________________ 6. ____________________

7. ____________________ 8. ____________________

9. ____________________ 10. ____________________

11. ____________________ 12. ____________________

13. ____________________ 14. ____________________

15. ____________________ 16. ____________________

17. ____________________ 18. ____________________

19. ____________________ 20. ____________________

21. ____________________ 22. ____________________

23. ____________________ 24. ____________________

25. ____________________

How can healthy eating help what you value the most?

1. ____________________ 2. ____________________

3. ____________________ 4. ____________________

5. ____________________ 6. ____________________

7. ____________________ 8. ____________________

9. ____________________ 10. ____________________

11. ____________________ 12. ____________________

13. ____________________ 14. ____________________

15. ____________________ 16. ____________________

17. ____________________ 18. ____________________

19. ____________________ 20. ____________________

21. ____________________ 22. ____________________

23. ____________________ 24. ____________________

25. ____________________

How will poor eating and avoiding exercise **hurt** what you value the most?

1. ______________________ 2. ______________________

3. ______________________ 4. ______________________

5. ______________________ 6. ______________________

7. ______________________ 8. ______________________

9. ______________________ 10. ______________________

Once you do this exercise, you'll never fall off the wagon. Healthy living will become one of your highest values. I can't stress enough how important this is. You will always work for what you value, and values can change.

Take the average college guy, for example. He cleans himself up, goes from party to party drinking all night, gets next to no sleep, and then wakes up and does it again. And he does this week after week. That's a lot of work!! That takes a lot of dedication and discipline. How is he able to continue doing that? For many guys in that stage of life, meeting girls is one of their highest values.

If you judged my level of discipline based on my ability to go partying all night, you'd think I was the laziest, most undisciplined person alive. It's not something I value and not something I'm willing to put effort into. The health of my family, on the other hand, is massively important to me which makes it easy to make healthful decisions.

As I'm writing this section, I just received this email:

"Hey Dr. Czys!! "Hope all is well with you! I just had to share...My daughter came home from school and was so proud of herself for improving her PACER test* by 10 seconds from last year. She said, 'Mom, I was the only girl left! I outran the last 3 boys!'

"She now comes into the gym with me and loves to do plank challenges, or anything that a nine-year-old is allowed to do in the gym. She shows me her biceps and says, 'Check this out!'

"I hope you know how grateful we are for what you do. This changes lives and allows us as parents to change our children's lives and prepare them for the future. From the bottom of my heart, thank you Steve! I couldn't ask for more as a mom."

That is why I do what I do!

*The PACER test is a fitness test: Progressive Aerobic Cardiovascular Endurance Run.

The Funk Doesn't Discriminate

You need to keep the list you created for when the FUNK happens. **The funk happens to everybody, it doesn't discriminate.** Sometimes when you're in a funk, you don't feel like doing much and your motivation is low. It happens to me and it's annoying; but I have my list. I just go back to my list and remind myself why I do what I do, and it re-motivates me and gets me out of the funk. Then I get in a good workout on top of that and feel amazing.

This is the most powerful technique I've found for sticking with a program. Please take the time to do it. Fill out all 50 reasons. If you have kids, I recommend placing their picture(s) on the table as you're filling them out. It's powerful, it's valuable, and it's worth your time.

GOALS: HOW TO INCREASE YOUR CHANCE FOR SUCCESS BY 77%

I'm sure you've heard the advice that you should write down your goals. Everyone has heard it. There are other ways to drastically increase the success rate of your goals for the short and long term as well. One way is to set the bar low and make it achievable: "I'm going to follow Dr. Czys' plan and lose two pounds this week." Set a goal, hit it, feel good and now you're ready to hit another goal. Set another one: small, achievable; and hit it. Those little goals build on each other, and compound into massive improvements.

Write your goals down at the end of this chapter and be specific. "I will start every day with the healthy fats and proteins Dr. Czys recommends," or "I will get an average of seven to nine hours of sleep per night," or "I will exercise for 30 minutes, 4 times per week." Make the goals easy and keep achieving them.

I need to insert a warning right here. Scales LIE! Often, you may lose fat—which is awesome—and gain muscle density, which is even more awesome. Dense muscle is heavy which means your body composition and health is drastically improving, but the scale hasn't changed! I've seen this hundreds of times: pants are falling down, cheekbones are more defined, and clothes are falling off, but the scale is showing the same number. It's lying to you! Just be aware of this!

If you have specific goals and you write them down where you can see them, your chance of success goes up about 40 percent. That's a pretty big increase in success, so I definitely recommend it!

Now, if you tell people close to you about your goals and when you plan to reach them, it gets even better. If you tell people your specific goals, it subconsciously keeps you more accountable and your chances of success go up by 77 percent! That's huge. Write down specific goals, make them public and tell others what your goals are and what you're working towards, and your likelihood of success increases by 77 percent. That's pretty freaking amazing. Do it! Another warning I'm adding is to say that people are inherently negative. Expect doubters when you tell them your goals. Use that as motivation! Prove them wrong!

Set the bar low repeatedly. A lot of small wins is much better than a big loss. If you set a goal of losing two pounds in a week, that is very achievable. When you set that goal and hit it, it's a win and you feel good. Set another goal to lose two pounds the next week, hit it, and win again. Those wins feel great and compound very quickly. Setting a goal to lose 50 pounds in 12 weeks is much more daunting. You could lose 40 which would be remarkable but if you fall short of the 50, it will feel like a loss. Set the bar low, crush it and keep crushing goals!

Here's one more trick that works for me: Wisdom. I like to think I'm wise when it comes to making choices about health. The wisest people throughout history have always made decisions based on long-term thinking. The unwise choice involves short-term thinking or immediate gratification. Far too often, people make decisions in favor of short-term pleasure, which almost always leads to greater long-term PAIN. An example is wanting a car now that you really can't afford. But you may really want the new car and think you need it. So, you may take out a loan and buy the car now even though you can't afford it. That $30,000 car becomes a $36,000 car after added interest. This would not be a wise purchase as you would just be giving away $6000 plus paying more for insurance every month. Unwise decisions involving our health have even worse consequences.

Crazy Statistic – On average, 52% of our income goes to taxes and 35% of post-tax income goes to interest! Another example of results from focusing on immediate gratification instead of thinking long term.

Too often, we choose a meal based on how we feel at that moment. This is short-term thinking. The pizza and beer will taste amazing for a few short moments. This choice is based on very short-lasting, immediate pleasure. We're not thinking about how terrible we'll feel later, or the gut rot, or feeling sluggish the next day, or that it's packing fat in all the wrong places and destroying our digestive system. We're not thinking about how much exercise it will take to burn off that one garbage meal or how the future pain is much greater than that one little short-term pleasure decision.

I always try and focus on the long term. So, when it comes to meal choice, I always think about how I will feel later in the day or the next day. Long-term thinking will benefit your health AND wealth! Your health will improve, and your bank account will grow!

It's so much easier to choose healthy when you're thinking long term. What's really cool is when you do this consistently and it becomes a part of who you are, the pleasure becomes both long AND short term. You can eat whatever the hell you want, but you CHOOSE healthy because that's who you are.

For a very long time, I was just like everyone else. I was raised eating crappy foods and drinking soda and all kinds of unhealthy stuff and I developed a taste for it. But now I've gotten to the point where I gain just as much pleasure from having a veggie stir fry or grilled chicken thighs or a piece of watermelon as I would if I ate a cookie, cake, chips, waffles, pizza or anything else that many people eat for pleasure.

Always come back to review this chapter because it doesn't matter what the plan is if you don't STICK with the plan. **Consistency is the most important aspect of any plan. You must understand that half-assed effort doesn't achieve half the results, it achieves little to NO results.** You must go all in and be consistent, and that's when the magic happens and how you'll reach your ultimate goal.

Future Pacing

There's power in future pacing: taking the time to visualize the future. Visualize six months or one year from now. If you apply what's in the book and stay consistent, in six months to a year you'll be exactly where you **want** to be. Visualize how good you're going to feel. You're buying new clothes that fit better. You have more energy. You're confident entering a room of people. You feel and look so much better.

OR the reverse happens. You don't apply what the book teaches. And instead of staying at the same level of health you're at now, you probably get worse. You put on an extra 20 pounds. You have to go buy new clothes again, but they're actually bigger clothes. You feel worse. It's harder to move. You're achier and have even less energy.

Here's the truth: Never, not one time, has a person applied what I teach and not achieved great results. You won't be the first because it's impossible. This will work for you! I guarantee it. Here's how I know it's going to work for you: because we're human. You and I are 99.5% genetically identical. All of us are, as members of the human species. Later in the book I will explain why that's so powerful. For now, just know this will work for you! Visualize your healthier future and apply what you read.

"The work of the doctor will, in the future, be ever more that of an educator, and ever less that of a man who treats ailments." – Sir Thomas J. Horder of Ashford (1871-1955), physician to several British monarchs.

Specific Goals:

____

Chapter 3: Take Control!

Dangers in Disguise

Raise your hand if you want to be healthy. Go ahead, raise your hand. I know, I know, you're sitting behind a book, and it feels kind of weird. Do it anyhow. You want to be healthy, right? Maybe you're in a coffee shop: just raise it anyway. People will be wondering, "What the hell? Is she asking a question? Does she want me to answer a question? Is she airing out her armpit?" Who cares what strangers think! But raise your hand if you want to be healthy. Or just nod your head yes, "Yes, I want to be healthy." Of course you want to be healthy. Healthy feels better and looks better. When someone loses their health, the only thing in the world they want is to get it back.

If I could snap my fingers and make you healthier, would you want me to do it? Of course you would. You didn't wake up this morning thinking you're just too damn healthy, did you? You didn't wake up thinking, "Man, I'm just too damn healthy. I better have a cigarette today to bring this perfect health down a notch." You want to be healthier. Unfortunately, I can't just snap my fingers to make it happen. I can, however, give you all the tools you need to make it happen; the tools you need to make it as easy and painless as possible!

Let me ask you this: Is there anything more important than your health? Think about it. Is there anything more important than your health (other than your kids' health)? Money? Your house? Your car? If you were dying, would you give up every penny you had to be healthy? Absolutely. What happens all the time is people paying whatever it costs to try and get back the health they lost because of consistent poor choices. Again, I must stress, there's nothing more important than your health, right? Yes. Nod your head, yes.

So, what's healthier, an apple or a doughnut? What's healthier, soda or water? It's an easy question. You know which one is healthier. Why do you still eat doughnuts? Why do you still drink soda? Why in the hell do we do that? We just agreed that nothing is more important than our health, yet we consistently make choices we know are bad for our health. Is it because that doughnut tastes so good?

Crazy Fact: Coca-Cola began as a pharmaceutical product.

Although most people would agree health is the most important thing, we frequently choose unhealthy food and drink. Why? What if I took that doughnut and put poison in it? Poison you couldn't taste or smell. Maybe it'll be the best tasting doughnut you've ever eaten. But in a week, it will kill you. Would you still eat the doughnut? Of course not, it's poison. What a stupid question. There's no way I'm going to eat that doughnut. Here's the thing, though: that doughnut, it IS poison. For Sure. That soda? It's poison. For Sure. But it takes decades to slowly poison and kill you, not a week.

One of the major goals of this book is to help you to understand the foods that many people commonly eat, and the foods that we often feed our children, are truly poison. They're just a slow-acting poison that's killing you over a long period of time. Once you realize this, once you see that doughnut as toxic, destroying your cells, ruining your joints, and ruining your brain, your mindset shifts to "Why would I ever eat that?", no matter how good it might taste.

I view a doughnut or a bottle of soda as if it were a cigarette. Think about it. Does a cigarette provide any health benefit? No. Does it provide anything other than short-term pleasure? No. Smoking is a nasty, expensive habit that destroys cells and causes cancer.

Consider a can of soda. Does it offer any health benefit? No. Does it give you anything other than short-term pleasure? No. Consistently drinking soda promotes cancer, arthritis, obesity, heart disease, diabetes, strokes, and much more. How can that be labeled anything but poison? Yet, kids drink it every day and nobody bats an eye. That's the power of marketing!

Really stop and think about how crazy this is. If you saw a person who was hooked up to an oxygen tank that allowed them to breathe, smoking, would you wonder, "What the hell?" Undoubtedly. Next, visit a public pool and you'll likely see many, many obese kids drinking soda and eating ice cream, while nobody appears concerned. How is that possible? Because so many people just don't view those foods as the poisons they truly are. A recent study has shown that poor diet is killing more people globally than smoking. That's how bad much of the food we eat and feed our families is (Afshin, et al. 2019).

Marketing convinces people to see doughnuts and soda and believe it's just "people food." What is this "people food?" What is this magic food that is okay for people yet bad for every other mammal? There's no such thing.

I've heard parents saying this sort of thing to their little kids. A child had a bag of chips and was trying to give some to the family dog, then his mother told him, "Oh gosh no honey, that's bad for the dog." What the shit? How is a bag of chips bad for a dog but okay for a child? It's because of the common belief system that says that chips and other junk food is people food and is okay for us to eat. We believe we are some super species and that the laws of physiology that apply to every other mammal somehow don't apply to us. That's just not true.

Whenever I talk to groups of kids, I ask them, "If you had a puppy, would you want it to feel loved, safe, and appreciated? Would you want the puppy to be healthy?" The kids always reply with an emphatic, "Yes!" Next, I ask them, "Would you feed the puppy really healthy food and really clean water?" They reply, "Absolutely, yes!"

What would happen if, for breakfast, we started that puppy off with cereal, pancakes, waffles, a muffin, or a pop tart along with juice instead of water? And then for lunch, we gave them a peanut butter and jelly sandwich with a juice box? And finally, for supper, we fed them pizza and Kool-Aid? It would undoubtedly make that dog sick. And this kind of diet is making us sick too.

There are a lot of foods you eat every day that you know are unhealthy, and you know you shouldn't be eating them, but you still do. I believe it's because you just don't realize *how* bad they are. It's far worse than you know and by the end of the book, you'll understand exactly why. Knowing this will make it so much easier to make better choices!

Telling people the dangers of smoking has been the greatest medical contribution in the past 60 years. Eliminating sugary drinks would have an even greater impact on people's health.

We Don't Appreciate It until It's Gone

"My favorite things in life don't cost any money. It's really clear that the most precious resource we all have is time." – Steve Jobs

I want you to imagine someone who is going through cancer treatment. The chemotherapy and radiation are costing tens if not hundreds of thousands of dollars. They feel miserable, they're in agonizing pain, puking all day, losing their hair, have very little energy and a low quality of life. They're hoping that the chemo and radiation kills the cancer before it kills them. Unfortunately, most of us have watched others experience this first hand.

Ask yourself, what is every person in this situation trying to gain more of? **Time!** They're paying a fortune and going through hell with the hope of buying more time.

What's the most valuable asset we have? Time. What really matters is not just time to exist but time with loved ones. Active time. Experiencing things in life with others. The most precious asset we have is time. What I'm going teach you will not only give you more time, but a much higher quality of time. Regrettably, many people don't understand the value of time until it's almost gone.

What are your fondest memories? Go ahead and think back. What memories stand out to you? Every single one of them is of an experience, isn't it? Not a single one is of a product you purchased.

You will not only gain more time; you will gain higher-quality time which will allow you to enjoy many more experiences and form many more great memories.

"He who gains time gains everything." – Benjamin Disraeli

Why "Getting Old Sucks" Is a Lie You Have Been Taught

"I have learned to seek my happiness by limiting my desires, rather than in attempting to satisfy them." – John Stuart Mill

When a baby is born, its autonomy (ability to take care of itself) is at zero. Without around-the-clock attention, that baby will die. But as the child gets older, his function begins to improve. He learns to sit up, then crawl, then walk, and over time, the baby's function increases. That child's function should continue to increase until he reaches a human's peak ability which is at about the age of 28 to 30. We should maintain a very high level of function until about 40 years old when Father Time starts to reduce it by about one percent per year.

Our function begins to slowly decrease over time, and we slow down a little bit. We're still dancing, hiking, and playing with our grandkids well into our eighties, nineties, and even at 100. And then at 115 years old one night, we just fall asleep and don't wake up.

At least, that's what is *supposed* to happen. In certain parts of the world called blue zones, first identified as such by Dan Buettner, this is common. People in blue zones commonly live an active, functional, enjoyable life well into their early hundreds.

But here's what typically happens: People's choices are so unhealthy, that it's common to see *teenagers* lose function. Many people in their twenties are having a hard time getting in and out of a car; stairs are exhausting for them, the thought of hiking up a hill is daunting, and they're fatigued throughout the day. Function quickly decreases and they can no longer play with their kids. They're on the side watching. Function continues to slide and on average, by 64, they can no longer take care of themselves. At 64! Now they are back to infancy stage. The next 10-20 years are spent in a nursing home. Those poor choices lead not only to loss of time, but loss of quality of life during the time remaining. The worst part of this story is that people in these nursing homes are full of regret. That is my biggest fear: nearing the end and regretting the choices I've made.

This scenario is what prompts people to say dumb shit like, "Getting old sucks," or "I don't want to get old, anyhow." It's because we visualize

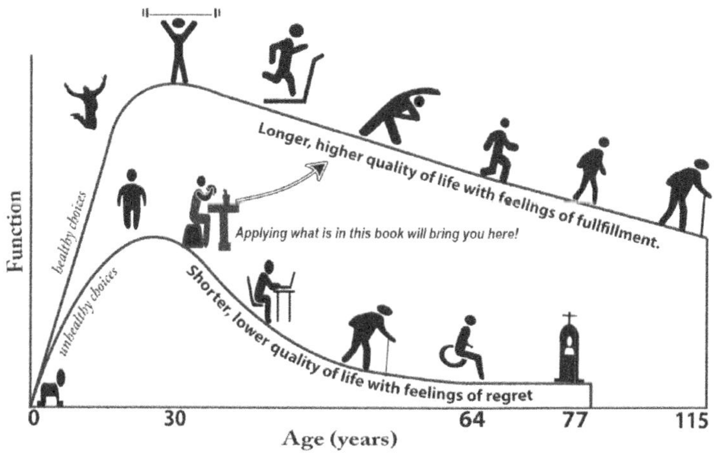

that second scenario as inevitable. It's not!

Wherever you are in your life, you can shoot up to the path of no regret! You will not only gain far more of your most important asset, time, you will gain a much higher quality of life during that time! I want to die with pride and satisfaction in my life.

By applying what's in this book, you will secure more quality time. Once you understand that cutting out that doughnut, soda, and chips, cutting out those foods that you know you shouldn't eat gives you more quality time with the people you love, making the right choices becomes easier. You'll get to ADD so many great foods in place of the junk. It will taste better, make you look and feel better, and help you live better. You'll not really be cutting things out as much as you will be adding delicious, healthy food into your life!

I will show you how powerful exercise truly is, how simple it is and how little time it really takes if you exercise properly. You can do this in less than two hours a week and build a great physique. You read that right. Less than two hours per week! The best part is that it won't include any time spent on boring cardio machines (hamster wheels)!

This will not only give you more time—decades more time—but higher quality, higher functioning time. Exercise is addicting, and you're going to fall in love with it. It will become so deeply ingrained in your brain that you will not be able to stop.

Right at the start of our lives, somebody should tell us that we are dying. Then we might live life to the limit, every minute of every day. Do it! Whatever you want to do, do it now. There are only so many tomorrows.

WHY THE STORY OF BAD GENES STEALS HOPE

Here is one of most tragic scenarios: We eat the doughnut. We drink the soda. We don't exercise. We don't get enough sleep. We poison ourselves with foods we shouldn't be eating. We feel like crap and go to the doctor. The doctor performs an exam and orders some blood work. He finds that you have high cholesterol, high blood sugar, high blood pressure and are overweight. He then asks about your family. Your mom and dad have had similar issues, as well as a couple of the grandparents, but that is as far back as you know. The doc then concludes, "Well, it must be genetic. Here, take these pills." **This is absolutely tragic.** Why? Because it takes away HOPE!

If you believe that you're overweight, sick and tired because you have bad genes, what do you hope to gain by changing? Why would you stop eating the doughnut if you think your health issues are from bad genes? You can't change your genes. Here is the great news: That doctor is completely wrong. Your situation is not the result of having bad genes. In fact, the bad choices have *changed* your genetic expression.

Allow Me to Explain How Flipping Amazing You Are!

Think about the special night when your mom and dad got in the back seat of a car and made you (sorry about that visual). In one special moment, you were created. You started off as one cell in your mother's womb with one set of genes, half from mom and half from dad. That one cell then made a copy of itself to become 2 cells, then 4, then 8, 16, 32 and so on. Those cells continued to duplicate, multiplying into about 75 trillion cells that equal YOU! Every one of those cells has the exact same genes. The best scientists in the world can't create one living cell. Your mother's womb created about 8,000 cells per second!

You have eye cells, hair cells, skin cells, muscle cells, liver cells, and about 200 different types of cells in your body. There are cells in your stomach that produce an acid that can dissolve a razor blade! Those acid-producing stomach cells have the same gene code as your eye cells, and every other cell. You have cells that break down the food you eat, and other cells use that digested food to build you. Every single cell in your body is produced from what you or your mother ate. All of those cells are made in the perfect order, in the perfect place, all from one set of genes in one cell. Is your mind blown yet? It will be, because you are amazing!

If I took the blood vessels out of you right now and lined them up, end to end, they'd go around the world twice. If I took the DNA out of your cells and lined it up. it would go around Pluto and back, twice! It's astonishing. Hundreds of trillions of chemical reactions happen every second within your body. How much is a trillion? If you go back in time one million seconds, that equals about 12 days. Go back in time one *trillion* seconds, and that equals 32,000 YEARS! You started as one cell and are now about 75 trillion cells, constantly working to keep you alive.

There is some type of intelligence within us, organizing hundreds of trillions of reactions within our cells every second of the day. I call this our innate intelligence, or intelligence within. Remember this innate intelligence—we'll come back to it soon.

I want you to visualize the most beautiful and perfect house that you could picture. This house has everything you could possibly want. Ladies, I know you've already done this! Visualize this perfect house. Can you see it? Excellent. We now have a blueprint to build this perfect home!

Now we need a construction crew. Imagine you've hired a construction crew that has never made a mistake. Their record is perfect. You have the perfect construction crew with the perfect blueprint to build the most perfect house. It's going to be flawless!

You've found the perfect location. Everything's ready, and you start ordering materials for the construction crew. The materials start to arrive and many of them are great, but you start receiving bent nails and a few broken windows, then some materials just never show up. Electrical wiring arrives, but not nearly enough. Yet some other materials just keep coming. You're getting way too many shipments of wood and it's just piling up and taking up space.

Could that amazing construction crew still put a house together for you? Absolutely. Would it match the blueprint perfectly? No. Would it function as well as it could? Absolutely not. Is it the blueprint's fault? No. Is it the construction crew's fault? No. It's the fault of the material. Let me explain why this is important.

What's your gene code? Your gene code is just a blueprint. Your gene code is the blueprint with directions how to build all 200 different types of cells in your body. And that innate intelligence I described earlier is the construction crew. The intelligence utilizes the materials you deliver and builds you. Where do the materials come from? From what you eat! An unhealthy, overweight body is almost *never* the fault of our genes, it's the fault of the materials, the foods we're giving our genes to work with. What matters are our choices and thankfully, we can change our choices! Obviously, some genetic diseases, i.e., Down syndrome, sickle cell anemia, etc. affect a certain percentage of individuals. However, the overwhelming majority of diseases are NOT genetic. There is NO such thing as an overweight or obesity gene!

The problem is that when we give our genes bad materials to work with, our innate intelligence is unable to create an amazingly healthy human body. We can't build that amazing home. So, here's the beautiful fact about this: You can change genetic expression based on the lifestyle choices you make! You *can* get lean! You *can* get toned! You *can* have more energy! You *can* feel amazing! I'll teach you how to give your body the absolutely best materials!

This fact is so important and so powerful. It gives us hope because no matter where any of us are at, we can improve, drastically. Even if a person has a genetic variant, this program will still benefit them. A person with Down syndrome will be far healthier if they eat healthful foods and exercise too!

This field of study is called epigenetics and explores how our choices turn genes on and off and can change genetic expression. Here is a simple example. Right now, I have hard calluses all over my hands. My skin is thicker and stronger than skin of most men my age. Is that a genetic defect? Or is that my body's response to weight lifting? Is it an epigenetic change?

If I quit exercising, started eating nothing but junk food, and complained all day, would I get fatter? Would my muscles disappear? Would my blood sugar and cholesterol go up? Absolutely. Would my high blood sugar and high cholesterol be the fault of bad genes? Of course not. They would be caused by bad choices. According to research, less than three percent of all illnesses can be attributed to a hereditary genetic cause.

Conclusive, related studies from Scandinavia followed identical twins throughout their lives. Identical twins have the exact same gene code. The twins in these studies grew up living different lifestyles and experienced massively different health outcomes even though they started with the same genes. How did they manage to look and feel so different while possessing the same gene code? Because they lived different lifestyles! They ate differently. They exercised differently. Their lifestyles significantly affected their genetic expression. It is so, so important that you understand this (Lichtenstein, et al. 2000).

It's crucial for you to understand that there's no such thing as an obesity gene. There's no gene that guarantees obesity. This fact is phenomenal because no matter what condition your body is in, when you change and follow this plan, you can become leaner, lose fat, feel better, have more energy and get the body you want. It's 100 percent, absolutely possible. We just have to maximize your genetic potential through the right choices.

One fact that I have always found interesting is that there IS actually a hangover gene. Is it possible to get a hangover without drinking? Of course not. Some people have a genetic variant that does not allow their body to produce the chemical that causes hangovers. Therefore, they would never get a hangover. For the rest of us, we experience hangovers. But we can only get them if we drink alcohol. Are hangovers a gene problem? Of course not. To prevent them, just don't overdrink. Thankfully, most things are not gene problems. They are the product of poor choices. It's time to start making the right choices!

Chapter 4: Mastering the Mentality and Psychology of Permanent Weight Loss

Statistics You Won't Believe Are True

So, how bad is it? Some of these numbers are mind blowing. For example, 62 million Americans, up to half of all adults, suffer from chronic gastrointestinal disorders. I find it unbelievable that this receives next to no media attention.

Do you think what we eat has an impact on how our digestive system feels? Absolutely. It's crazy to think that half of all adults are suffering. So, what are we doing? We're taking antacids and acid blockers. We spend about $7 BILLION a year on prescription and over-the-counter products to relieve indigestion. I'm sure you've seen the commercials on TV: Some guy is sitting at the deli counter ordering a burger, fries and a soda. He stops and rubs his belly because his acid reflux is kicking in. We're eating such terrible foods that our body is rejecting it. This burning feeling, this symptom is our body's way of telling us to change what we're shoving into our stomachs. So, what do we do? We take an acid blocker. Instead of fixing the problem, we block that symptom with a pill and continue eating the foods that are causing the problem.

Colon cancer is the second leading cause of cancer deaths in the US, killing more people every year than breast cancer. Your colon is your large intestine. Do you think what you eat and the food sitting in your colon has an impact on the health of your colon? Absolutely! What you eat has a huge impact. We aren't born with a cancerous colon. Both the unhealthy food and the lack of good food causes damage to our colon. I have worked with people who were literally already scheduled to have sections of their intestines removed, showed them how to eat, and have watched them heal! That's how powerful food is!

Speaking of cancer, on average, half of men and one third of women in the US and UK are predicted to develop cancer (Ahmad, Ormiston-Smith and Sasieni 2015). That's terrifying and the truth is that very few cancers are genetic. Only about five percent of cancers can be attributed to genetic defects. The remaining 95 percent have their roots in the environment and lifestyle, most of which are under our control! In May 2018, a report from the World Cancer Research Fund linked 12 types of cancers, including breast and colorectal, to being overweight (World Cancer Research Fund 2018). You can drastically reduce your chances of getting cancer just by following the advice in this book.

Unfortunately, most of us have been touched by cancer in some way. A family member, a friend, ourselves. It's so common. One of the most unfortunate things about it is this belief system that it's genetic. If we believe it's because of bad genes and our choices don't matter, we are less likely to make good choices.

One particular study that I really found fascinating showed that adopted children whose parents got cancer were much more likely to get cancer as well. So, even though the kids had no genetic link whatsoever, their chances of getting cancer went way up. Why? Because they were living in the same environment as their adoptive parents! They had the same lifestyle. They followed the same diet pattern and habits as their parents (Sørensen, et al. 1988). A huge percentage of cancers can be reduced just by following the advice in this book. Most types of cancer are a preventable disease!

Right now, the obesity numbers are staggering. According to the CDC, over 75 to 80 percent of Americans are overweight and 40 percent are considered obese (Prevention 2016). Our kids are fatter than they've ever been in history. Childhood obesity has tripled in the past 20 years. One in three kids eats fast food every single day. Forty percent of kids born between 2000 and 2011 will develop diabetes. Think about that. Two out of five kids will develop diabetes? Why? Could that drastic increase possibly be because of bad genetics? What is the solution we are being sold? Drugs. Spending in 2018 for diabetes drugs in the US reached $53.7 billion last year, more than double what was spent in 2013. In about four years, spending on diabetes medications increased by $27 billion dollars. Just to be clear, I'm only talking about type 2 diabetes which used to be called adult onset diabetes. However, it has become so common in children, the name was changed to type 2 diabetes. Or, lifestyle diabetes.

People commonly commit suicide via lifestyle. Our choices are slowly killing us and our kids.

When you look at the chart below, the numbers are scary. And it's worse than it looks. These rates are based on BMI or Body Mass Index. The BMI is actually a useless number as it doesn't factor in muscle. I am very lean, but my BMI says I'm obese. However, many women have what is considered a "healthy" BMI but are overweight or obese. Body fat percentage is a much more accurate number and the rates are even worse. About 80 percent of people in the US are overweight and our kids our getting heavier and heavier at younger ages.

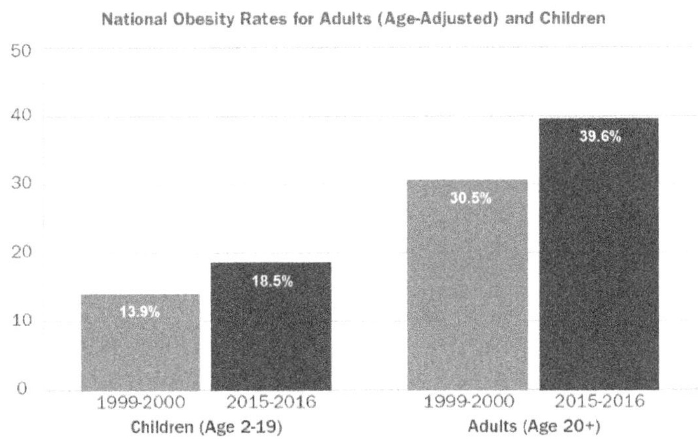

Source: CDC

"You're going to give him/her an eating disorder!" We've all heard this before. I have to address this now and it's something you can share with any misinformed family members. It's amazing how many times I've had parents make the wise transition to healthier foods only to get push back from family members. "You're going to give him/her an eating disorder!" says Grandma.

How in the hell can providing healthy food for your child give them an eating disorder? That's like giving your kid cigarettes so they won't smoke later in life. How does feeding a child chronic-disease-causing junk food prevent an eating disorder? Do you really think there is a single person out there that has an eating disorder because he/she didn't eat enough junk food as a child? That is how powerful marketing is! It perpetuates that much ignorance.

Love Your Body and Eat for Health

The key to doing it right is to instill the value of health in your kids. Teach them to love and appreciate their amazing bodies and to feed and fuel their bodies with great tasting, healthy foods.

The problem arises when we use words like "skinny" as a positive. When people strive for skinny, they don't care about health and make poor choices just to achieve skinny. When you eat for health and you enjoy a bowl of berries as much as candy, you'll be lean and healthy without ever trying to be skinny.

We need to teach kids and ourselves not to compare our lives to fake lives. On Instagram and other social media, personalities look so happy, so gorgeous (with their filters after 50 takes in perfect lighting) and we compare ourselves, making us feel worse. We have no idea how unhappy that person may be. Especially the ones who are so fake while deep down they have to live with their lying selves.

"Comparison is the thief of joy." – Theodore Roosevelt

Over half our kids are overweight and each year more kids are found to have heart disease, diabetes, asthma, allergies and attention-deficit disorder issues. In fact, atherosclerosis—the beginning signs of heart disease—is now commonplace in kids. Read that paragraph again.

More than two thirds of the adult population is either overweight or obese. There was a 600 percent increase in just 15 years. Could these drastic increases possibly be the result of bad genes? Absolutely not. It's the result of bad choices. And the good news about this is that there is hope. We can change our choices and quickly reverse this trend.

For example, a nurse's health study showed that not smoking, walking, and maintaining a healthy body weight reduced the risk of diabetes by over 90 percent (Kott and Fruh 2009). I'm going to show you how easy it is and give you step-by-step tools to show exactly how to do it. But first, we need to discuss prescription drug use.

Crazy Fact – Merck (pharmaceutical company) knew that Vioxx (arthritis medication) increased heart attack risk. The FDA estimated its use caused 90,000-140,000 heart attacks. Merck paid out over $6 billion in settlements. However, they sold over $11 billion worth of product (The Washington Post Company 2004).

Problems Medication Can't Fix

First, I must say that clearly there are drugs that can and do save lives. Amazing medications have drastically helped me in a crisis. Some doctors or naturopaths think that some herbs or tonics will fix everything. But, that's just not true. The best medicine is an intelligent combination of proper lifestyle choices and nutrition and the proper use of medical intervention.

The US makes up less than five percent of the world's population; we're very small. Yet, we consume over HALF the medications on the planet. We're eating crap, much of what government tells us is healthy is completely Unhealthy, and we feel terrible. We go to the doctor and they are so quick to hand out pills. Amazing medications exist, but they will never fix a problem caused by poor lifestyle choices.

Eighty percent of American adults have a chronic illness! Examples of chronic illnesses are arthritis, obesity, high blood pressure, high cholesterol, and diabetes.

About 76 percent of Americans regularly take prescription drugs. On average, every person receives 11.2 prescriptions per year.

It gets worse. For seniors, it's 31 prescriptions per year.

And even worse, kids, on average, receive four prescriptions per year!

On average, Americans are consuming 50 million pills per hour. We are taking so many medications that scientists are now finding traces of medications in fish, frogs, shellfish and other water creatures. The medication in our urine is poisoning the environment!

So, what is this costing us? There are many debates on healthcare, but they never address the important question. All they debate is who should pay for health insurance. All they talk about is who should be paying for a broken system. Zero discussion about how to make people healthier!

How much is this broken system costing us?

Chronic Illness Costs
Heart disease and stroke - $545 million
Cancer - $477 million
Digestive disorders - $372 million
Obesity - $402 million
Diabetes - $649 million
Arthritis - $383 million
EVERY SINGLE DAY! $2.8 billion per day!
(Promotion 2019)

Chronic illness accounts for 78 percent of all healthcare spending, 99 percent of Medicare spending, and 83 percent of Medicaid spending.

According to the National Academy of Sciences, 30 percent of healthcare spending provides zero benefit. Healthcare WASTE costs $1.2 trillion per year or $2.4 million per minute.

As mind boggling as those numbers are, they don't include the cost of treatments dealing with side effects of medications. Properly prescribed medications are the leading cause of hospitalization and the fourth leading cause of death in the US.

Spending on prescription drugs has risen 600 percent since 1990 in the US.

In the US, prescription drug spending in 2002 had increased to 55 times as much as the spending in 1960 (Medicine 2010). If eggs and oranges increased at the same rate, eggs would cost about $50 a dozen, and a dozen oranges would cost about $134. In 2018, the US spent $943 million per day on retail medications, not including retail drug sales (Statista 2019).

The overwhelming majority of this spending is the result of poor diet! When you're looking at your insurance premiums and healthcare bills wondering why it's so ridiculously expensive, realize that this is caused by the terrible American lifestyle. This spending cannot be sustained. The projected growth will bankrupt the country.

The best-selling drug of all time, the cholesterol-lowering drug Lipitor, has not been shown to prevent heart disease or heart attacks!

I'm not done; amazingly, it gets worse. We're taking more medications than ever. We spend, by far, the most money in the world on healthcare per capita. By far! It's not even close. So, you would think that America is a pretty healthy country and we all live for a long time.

Life Expectancy

The US actually ranks fiftieth in life expectancy. Can you even name 49 countries? There are 49 countries where people live longer than we do. Even though we spend the most money on healthcare and take the most medications.

Think about it. Could that possibly be because in America, we just have bad genes? Where are most American relatives from? Those other countries where they live longer than we do! So, what happens when people come to America? Do their genes change? No, they just adopt the lifestyle of the typical American which, unfortunately, is not healthy. What is the life expectancy in the US? It's about 77 years old and has dropped the last 2 years! For the first time in history, our kids will average a shorter lifespan than their parents!

On average, women live two years longer than fellas. Why is that? Well the truth is, because women are smarter. I believe that 100 percent. My fitness facilities' and healthcare clients are about 75 percent female. Women value health more and are more likely to make healthy decisions. I'd bet money that the overwhelming majority of people reading this book are women. I want to add that I don't care what sex you are...I truly appreciate you! You clearly value health and that's awesome in my book!

Women also aren't as likely to do the dumb, risky things young guys do. Somehow, guys have been targeted by marketing to accept and even be proud of a beer gut, or a dickie-do (when your belly sticks out farther than your penis). Fellas, if you look down and can't see the little man, there's nothing cool about that.

What about functional life expectancy? In my opinion, life isn't life if you're strapped to a bed and you can't feed yourself. If you can't go to the bathroom on your own and you can't live without help, you've ridden the parabola back to infancy. What is the current functional life expectancy? 64 years old! Holy shit. Most people have big plans for retirement. But if they don't take care of themselves, when retirement comes, they don't have the health to enjoy it. I can't tell you how many patients I've worked with whose retirement consisted of going to various doctor appointments all the time.

I'll never forget a morbidly obese financial advisor who preached to me about planning for the future. All the money in the world wasn't going to fix his future. Your body is a hell of a lot more important than your bank account. Don't ever forget that. Nothing is more valuable than you are!

In the past 20 years, we've observed massive increases in chronic illness, sickness and disease in both middle-aged adults and children. You may be thinking, "Well, it's because the population is older and older people just get sicker and are prone to more disease." That's completely untrue because the fastest increase in disease and chronic illness has been in middle-aged adults and kids, not the elderly or the baby boomers. Each year for the past 50 years, Americans have spent more money per person on drugs and surgery to treat chronic illness. Each year for the past 50 years, chronic illness rates have risen. And every year for the past 50 years, death rates have risen as well. Epic fail.

After learning this, this is where wisdom comes into the picture, as I talked about earlier in the book. Wise people realize this and think long term and plan. They ask, "What do I want my future to be? Do I want to be stuck in a nursing home?" Unfortunately, this eventuality is so common that we believe that's the only possible outcome. But it's not!

What *should* happen is our sixties, seventies and eighties should be very active and fun just like our teen years, twenties and thirties should be! Many, many people out there have great lives in their eighties and nineties. They're active and driving and golfing and just living. They are having a great time. You can too. You just have to make the choice now.

Some people have responded to me or sent messages or commented on my Facebook page saying, "Oh, what difference does it make what you eat, we're all going to die eventually." Yes, we're all going to die eventually. However, when you live like crap, you're going to feel like crap, you're going to look like crap, and you're going to die earlier. It's not just the quantity that decreases, but also the quality. If this is true for you, you'll look back full of regret.

Make the decision now to change your choices. Change your lifestyle and think about the future. Think with wisdom. The short-term pleasures, treats, booze, cigarettes, poor foods and lack of exercise are going to ruin your future, and you will look back with regret. For me, there is nothing scarier than living with regret. If you've ever been to a nursing home, you've seen tons of people filled with regret. What's the number one regret people have on their deathbed? That they didn't live true to themselves. That they didn't live a good, healthy life. It's the number one regret. This is the time, no matter what situation you're in. You can choose the path of health and look and feel so much better and more importantly, your kids and others in your life are also going to look and feel so much better.

This is called the ripple effect. When you make better choices, the health and happiness of those around you improves. Your choices ripple to those around you. The longer you continue at it, the further and wider your ripple spreads. How can you get your family to change? Just quietly lead by example. Eventually they'll follow.

Health or excuses: you really have just two choices. You can choose health and vitality, energy and confidence, feeling and looking great, and the ability to buy and wear the clothes you like. Or you can do what most do and choose excuses. Everybody, and I mean everybody, gives me the exact same excuses. I've yet to meet a person that doesn't have any. Yet, some people choose action instead of excuses.

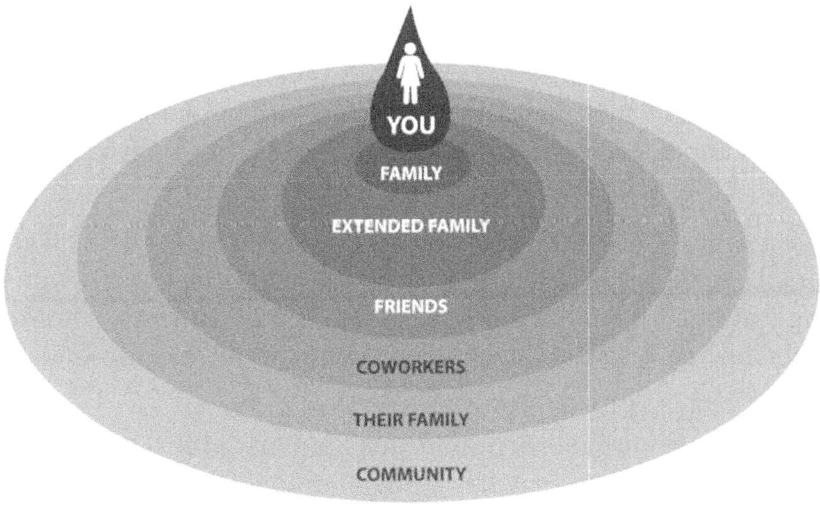

Everyone can say they're too busy. Everyone can say they can't afford it. Everyone can say they don't have time. Everyone can say this or that hurts. You can CHOOSE to not use those excuses and work towards being healthy. You need to decide what you want. Do you want health, vitality, a better appearance, confidence, to feel great, or do you want to make excuses?

"Time and health are two precious assets that we don't recognize and appreciate until they have been depleted." — Denis Waitley

The Great Healthcare Debate: Republicans Vs Democrats

The political nonsense in the media regarding healthcare drives me crazy. Neither side is talking about how to make America healthier. All I hear about is how to get more people insured, provide more people with drugs, and change who pays for this failing system.

They talk about access to cheaper meds, yet properly prescribed meds are the leading cause of hospitalizations and the FOURTH LEADING CAUSE OF DEATH IN THE UNITED STATES!

The debate is really about who should be paying for a failing system that costs more every year while people get sicker every year. Healthcare is actually sick care and is going to bankrupt the country.

Zero talk about how three fourths of Americans are overweight or how to solve that problem. Zero talk about how over one third of Americans have or will likely soon have diabetes. Zero talk about how childhood obesity has tripled in the past 20 years and HALF of American kids are overweight!

Why aren't they discussing how to make exercise a part of each school day for all ages? Discussing how to drastically improve school lunches? Talking about shutting down the food industry lobbyists (legalized bribery) so the government will stop promoting such awful eating advice?

The next time you are out in public, just stop and look around. Look at how many people are overweight, limping, hunched over, and unhealthy. Is that the result of poor insurance coverage? Or the result of poor lifestyle choices which usually begins at a very young age?

In our current healthcare system, less than three percent is spent on lifestyle and prevention. The majority of what is spent on "prevention" is for blood pressure screenings, cholesterol tests, blood sugar tests, etc. That's not prevention; that's early detection!

Eat like shit, don't exercise, develop symptoms, then go see a doctor covered by insurance to get some pills to mask those symptoms without a single conversation about what's causing them. That system is an epic failure.

Note: I'm not anti-med or anti-hospital; both obviously can and do save lives. However, diseases caused by poor lifestyles can never be fixed by a pill. Changing lifestyle choices is the only cure - not much money to be made from that.

The Price You Are Paying for Poor Policies

I want you to travel back in time with me. Let's travel back to when the United States Department of Agriculture (USDA) determined what the food groups were, and then established the food pyramid (Stuff 2018).

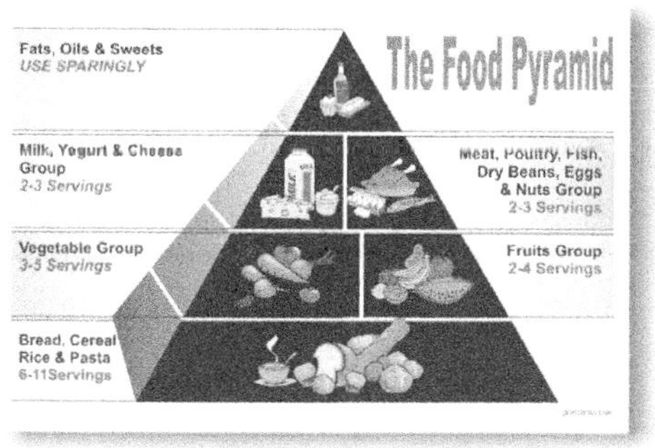

Visualize the USDA meeting where this advice originated from.

When you think of the USDA, do you visualize a group of healthy people sitting around a room asking the question, "How do we make Americans as healthy as possible?" Or do you see a group of men sitting in a room, asking the question, "How do we sell more of our country's agricultural products, such as corn, wheat, dairy and soybeans?" Which scenario makes more sense? Who was lobbying them? Were there lobbyists from the agriculture industry trying to lobby these people to sell agriculture products? Or were there people in healthcare trying to lobby them to teach Americans how to eat and be as healthy as humanly possible? There's far less money to be made off from healthy people!

For years, Barry Marshall and Robbi Warren were ridiculed for claiming bacteria can cause an ulcer. They even drank the bacteria and got an ulcer to prove it! Eventually, they won a Nobel prize (Weintraub 2010).

If you're old like me, you may remember that the biggest recommended part of the food pyramid, or the largest part of our diet was grains. Did that really make us healthy OR did the United States really want to sell those products? Over time, the USDA decided that the US food pyramid wasn't working very well so they came up with the food plate concept. One of the largest portions on the food plate is grains and instead of including a glass of water, a glass of milk is advised.

Why would that be? Was this because grains and dairy are required by humans to be healthy? Absolutely not! I'll explain why in detail soon. This plate guideline was influenced by lobbyists and money, not by science or logic. Lobbying is really just legalized bribery; let's call it what it is.

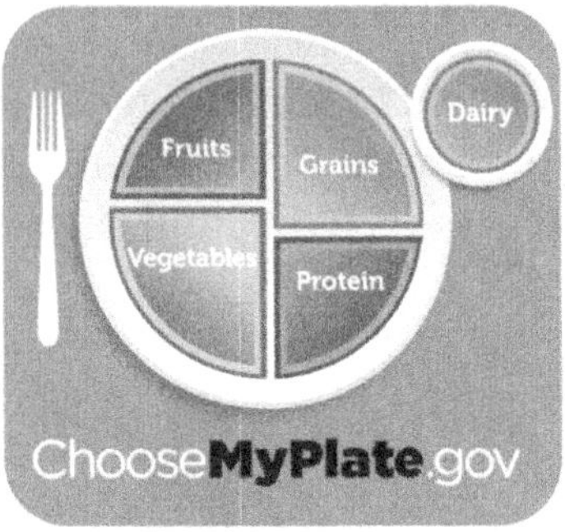

The first dietary guidelines published in 1980 were designed specifically to combat heart disease which was and still is public health enemy number one. These guidelines were partially based on studies that linked heart disease to sodium, cholesterol, and saturated fats. The problem was that these studies were seriously flawed and their *conclusions* incorrect.

Along with the flawed studies and incorrect conclusions came the FEAR of FAT! Be honest with me—have you ever bought something because the package said, "low fat?" Nod your head if you have. You've been in a store looking at options and thought, "Ooh, this one has low fat so it must be good for me and eating this means less fat *on* me." Why did you make that choice? Because years of marketing have conditioned you to believe fat is bad and eating low-fat foods is good for you.

What happens when you take fat out of food? It tastes like cardboard. What do food companies do to make you love it? They add a whole bunch of sugar. In the late 70s and early 80s, we were warned away from saturated fat and started eating all kinds of low-fat processed foods. Low-fat was plastered on just about everything. Instead of steak and eggs for breakfast, it was toast and jelly, cereal, waffles, pancakes, etc. Don't you dare put butter on that pancake but go ahead and bathe it in syrup.

Speaking of bullshit studies: About 50 years ago, the Sugar Research Foundation flat out paid researchers to create false study conclusions showing sugar was not a cause of heart disease but that fat was to blame instead (Kearns, Schmidt and Glantz 2016). One of the researchers was the chairman of Harvard's Public Health Nutrition Department. Today, Coca-Cola and a candy trade association are still trying the same tactics. A candy trade association funded and influenced studies to show that children who ate sweets had a healthier body weight than those who did not!

At the same time, the US government also started recommending "vegetable" oils because they were not saturated fats. One interesting fact about vegetables oils is they're not actually made from vegetables; they are made from grains and legumes. Canola oil, which is actually rape seed oil (the name was changed because "rape oil" wouldn't sell very well), and corn oil are from grains and soybean oil is from legumes.

These oils are terribly unhealthy as they damage your cells and the lining of your arteries, essentially, they damage you! This damage results in inflammation which results in hardening of the arteries and heart disease among many other health problems. These oils, especially when combined with refined grains, turn your body into a fat-storing machine! Not good.

If you drive anywhere around the Midwest, you will oceans of fields of corn and soybeans. The government uses tax dollars to pay farmers to grow these terribly unhealthy foods. This creates a mass abundance which makes it super cheap. And this is why you find high-fructose corn syrup, corn starch, and soybean oil in so many products. Corn is even used to make gasoline, allowing it to gunk up our engines as well as your arteries! How nice would it be if healthy organic foods were subsidized, which would bring the cost of quality food down?

Unfortunately, the current system just keeps getting worse. All of this corn, canola and soy are "Roundup-ready" crops (genetically altered to withstand the Roundup herbicide) so these oceans of corn and soy are sprayed year after year with Roundup. Roundup kills every single plant it touches other than the corn, canola and soy that has been genetically modified to be immune to the poison. Roundup from Monsanto, which was recently purchased by Bayer (drug company) for $66 billion, just lost a lawsuit showing Roundup caused cancer. They were served 8,000 new lawsuits the following week. That's certainly a good start towards fighting this insanity. Researchers have found cancer-causing Roundup in numerous cereals and other products commonly fed to kids. The good news is I'm about to show you how easy it is to avoid eating this awful product.

Corn is so cheap that giant grasslands are sprayed with Roundup which kills all vegetation and any bugs that feed on the grasses which also kills any birds that feed on the bugs or grass seeds. The dead grasslands are then plowed under, killing and destroying the habitat of any small mammals living in those grasslands. It's no wonder there are fewer birds, butterflies, and bees; fewer *everything* other than corn or soy. Corn is then planted, and a large portion of this corn is harvested and fed to cattle. All of that gas burning, poison spraying, and topsoil eroding to grow corn for cattle instead of just allowing cattle to graze on prairies.

I'll cover this in detail later, but corn-fed cattle are very unhealthy for human consumption. Grass-fed cow meat is actually very good for us. So, instead of allowing cattle to graze on the grasslands which is better for everything, farmers are spraying, plowing, and planting the same fields year after year after year. This practice is not sustainable and it's destroying our habitat. As the habitat goes, so too goes its inhabitants.

The environmental impact alone is devastating. I live among these oceans of Roundup-ready corn and soybean fields. These fields are more like deserts than oceans as there is very little life within them. It's really fascinating when you walk along these fields and come to hills that are a little too steep or areas the sprayers missed. Here, you'll find a large variety of grasses and flowers growing. About every three weeks, new varieties of gorgeous flowers begin to bloom. There are grasshoppers and other bugs everywhere, chipmunks and rabbits and birds and such a variety of sounds. It really sounds like a musical of bugs and birds singing. But in the corn and soy fields...silence. A manmade desert.

Never Forget: As the Habitat Goes, so Too Goes Its Inhabitants

Based on government advice, Americans started eating a wide variety of grains, more sugars, and grain oils, and since the late 70s, obesity and diabetes has absolutely skyrocketed. This was an epic failure and *still* many nutritionists, hospitals, and the American Heart Association keep recommending the same diet.

What you must understand is the government's eating advice is not based on science or logic. The goal of most politicians is to get elected and re-elected. They make policies to keep the contributors that give them money happy. Because of this corruption, the food and agriculture industries have far too much influence on government policies. This idea isn't some conspiracy theory craziness, it is fact.

Think about the history of government food advice. For 50 years, they told people to avoid eggs, one of the most nutrient-dense, amazing foods you can eat. For many years, intelligent people demonstrated exactly why that advice was wrong, and how it didn't make any sense. How eating cholesterol doesn't raise your body's cholesterol. Eighty percent of your cholesterol is produced by your body, by your liver. If you eat a bunch of cholesterol, your body will just make less. High cholesterol is largely a result of the grains and grain oils your government tells you is "heart healthy."

I start almost every day with six eggs. As I mentioned, for 50 years, the government told people to avoid eggs, and eat cereal instead. Organizations such as the American Heart Association recommend you eat Cheerios instead of an egg or avocado. The AHA literally recommends low-fat Pop Tarts over eating salmon, because salmon has fat in it and a Pop Tart doesn't (Lilburn 2016). This advice is so dumb that it's almost laughable, yet people not only follow it, but teach it!

Remember when the government recommended eating margarine and not eating saturated fat? The government gave nutrition advice that was so bad, it killed hundreds of thousands of people and trans-fats are still in many of the foods people feed kids every day. They're so toxic, the World Health Organization is trying to ban trans-fats altogether.

How can government food advice be so bad? Again, because the officials in charge of this have been bought.

$6 billion is spent every year on bariatric surgery (weight-loss surgery) in the US. On average, after one year, 4.6 percent of those patients DIE (Schauer, et al. 2010).

Why Are Most Diet Plans Wrong? They Ask This Question, and It's Wrong

"The only thing you should ever replace a meal with is a healthier meal!" Dr. Czys

It's no secret Americans have been gaining weight at a rapid pace for a long time. Our kids are heavier than they've ever been, and anywhere our Western culture spreads to, the people very quickly start gaining weight too. Countless diet plans, pills, cleanses and detox products have been sold to try and combat the issue. The problem with almost all plans is they ask the wrong question. They ask, "What should a person do to lose weight?" The correct question is, **"What is the optimal diet for humans?"** When you ask how to lose weight, you will hear about all kinds of crazy diet plans that are terrible for health. I'll go over a few below. You might think I made them up, but they're all real!

Back in 1925, Lucky Strike cigarettes launched a campaign with the slogan, "Reach for a Lucky Instead of a Sweet." I'm not going to lie: if you decide to smoke instead of eat, you will lose weight. It's just not the wisest approach to do so...

In 1977, SlimFast came out with "A shake for breakfast, a shake for lunch, and then a sensible dinner." Today, there are countless meal replacement shakes that are ridiculously overpriced and rarely good for you. Here's a fantastic rule scribed in stone: **The only thing you should ever replace a meal with is a healthier meal!** Don't worry, I'll show you how to do exactly that.

In the early 90s, Americans went for low-fat foods like the McDonald's McLean Deluxe burger, with a diet soda and jumbo fries! How well did that work out? There are dozens and dozens of examples like this because Americans ask the wrong question.

Before starting any diet plan, ask these questions: Would it make sense for a kid to follow this diet? Would you start counting calories for a kid? Would you ever consider putting a kid on a macro plan? Would you expect a child to try the Atkins Diet? The beauty of my eating program is that it makes sense for people of any age! This is the ONLY plan that makes sense.

Body-Wrapping an Overweight Dog

Numerous different cleanses, detoxes, 21- or 30-day challenges, body wraps, lasers and more promise quick fat loss. Visualize this scenario for me. Let's say your dog put on a bunch of extra fat and didn't move around much. That happens, right? Is it possible for a pet to eat too much unhealthy food and get fat? Absolutely. It's actually quite common. Let's say you took this overweight dog to the vet and the vet told you, "You know what this dog really needs? It really needs a 24-day detox and fat-burning pills." I'm sure you'd think to yourself, *That is the dumbest thing I've ever heard*...right? But humans do it all the time.

What if you took an overweight dog to the vet and the vet said, "You know what this dog needs? It just needs a good body wrapping. Body wrap the dog twice a day and the fat will melt away." That's absurd, isn't it? Yet people buy into this advice for themselves all the time. Not after this book. NEVER again!

Do you know what all of these cleanses, challenges, detoxes and body wraps have in common? Not a single one of them have a shred of evidence to support their claims! This would be a really easy study to conduct and yet NONE of the companies have done this. Simply gather two groups of people. One group is given an exercise and healthy eating program. Another group of is given the same exercise and healthy eating program along with whatever nonsense shake or cleansing product the company is trying to sell. Let them go at it for eight weeks and see which group does better. Then track their results for an extended period of time as well. If both groups are eating well and exercising, they'll both have great results!

Another option would be to take two groups of people and give each of them the same shake or cleanse program. Assign one group a diet and exercise program to follow as well, while the other group consumes the products without changing any diet or exercise habits. Why haven't these simple studies been done? There is a reason for including the phrase "along with a healthy diet and exercise" as part of these programs. That is the part that gives you the results!

The reason none of these studies have been done is because the companies that make these products aren't stupid. They're not going to perform a study that proves their products don't work. What they do instead is use very clever marketing. They use stories and emotion to sell. Marketing departments know that stories sell better than science and logic.

If this book accomplishes just one thing, and convinces you to NEVER buy the cleanse, detox, wraps or whatever your neighbor, friend or family member is pushing, I'm happy. Writing the book was worth the effort.

What about detoxes? Again, a very simple study would show whether they work or not. Test a person to find out which toxins are in their body. Give them the detox and then test them again to prove they are now less toxic. This has never been done! Why? Your kidneys, liver, lymphatic system, lungs, etc., are cleansing your body of toxins every second of the day.

Yet another option would be to give a person a detox drink, shake, or pills and then test their urine, sweat, feces, and breath for toxins being excreted. Again, this has never been done! Why? Because they know the products don't work!

Have you ever seen those ionic foot baths that claim to pull toxins from your feet? The water turns a rusty brown color and that is considered proof of the toxins pulled from your body. Guess what was found in the water when it was actually tested? Rust! No toxins—Ever!

We need to support our amazing detoxing organs with healthy foods and stop poisoning them with junk food. Let's talk about what you should and shouldn't choose, to be able to do exactly that.

Chapter 5: Why the Type of Macro You Eat (Carb, Fat, Protein) Is More Important Than the Amount of Macros

Good Carbs vs Bad Carbs - What Most Doctors and Nutritionists Don't Understand

Nutrition is actually quite simple. We just insist on making it complicated. There is absolutely no nutritional reason to eat grains and there are, as you're about to learn, many reasons to avoid them.

It's time to make choosing healthy foods really, really easy for you. I'm going to break it down by macronutrients (carbs, fats, and proteins) and make it so simple, it will almost be hard to believe.

Let's start with carbohydrates. Here's what I'd like you to do: Visualize a Lego block in each hand. If you have kids, go grab some Legos; seriously. Go grab some of the Legos you are constantly dancing around. Okay, now that you have a Lego in each hand, in one hand, you have a Lego that's called glucose, a simple sugar. In the other hand, you have another Lego, called fructose, which is another simple sugar. Take those Legos and put them together. Now you have sucrose, which is table sugar. Now I want you to add another Lego and boom! you have a carbohydrate. A carbohydrate is just sugars bound together.

Now keep adding Legos; add two, three, four or more until the shape starts to look a little more complex. This is a complex carbohydrate. All carbohydrates are just sugars bound together. The more sugars that are bound together in a carbohydrate, and the faster your body can digest or break them down, generally, the worse they are for you. Digestion happens when your body takes that carbohydrate and breaks it down into those individual Legos, into glucose and fructose, and eventually your body breaks that fructose into glucose. Your body uses that glucose for energy. When you consume too much, your body converts the sugar to fat and stores it.

The more sugars that are in a carbohydrate and the faster your body can break them down, the worse it is for you. Also, the lower that carbohydrate is in fiber and vitamins or minerals, the worse it is for you.

How do you make a cow gain weight really fast? You lock it up so it can't exercise, and you feed it corn. Why? Because corn is a grain and grains are basically just balls of sugar. I have to mention here that corn is NOT a vegetable! Corn-fed cattle very quickly put on hundreds of pounds of fat.

Recently, I read a story about a truck full of Skittles that crashed on the way to a farm in Wisconsin. Why Skittles? Because the farmer could buy expired candy cheaper than corn for his cattle, a less expensive form of sugar to fatten them up with. The real interesting reaction to me was the consumer outrage. "How could you feed Skittles to a cow?!" Skittles are marketed to kids every day and nobody says a thing about it. The reason candy is on shelves at kids' eye level and covered in cartoons is because manufacturers want your kids to see it and ask you for it. That should cause outrage!

The debate really isn't about whether or not grains are good or bad for humans. The debate is about marketing and money vs science and logic. I am constantly being asked, "How are grains bad for me?" What about asking, "How are grains *good* for me?" Most people already believe they are healthy. Why? Because that's what we have been persuaded to believe through marketing.

Let's first answer the question, how are grains good? Let me start by declaring that there is not a SINGLE nutrient found in grains that you won't consume more of when eating how I will teach you to. This is very important. There is nothing in grains you won't get more of from eating fruits, vegetables, nuts, meats, and eggs.

In fact, humans don't need to eat grains at all. If you examine human history, you'll find humans existed on virtually a grain-free diet for 1.7 million years. We only started eating grains during the agricultural revolution 10,000 years ago.

It's important to point out the grains of today are very different than they were even a couple hundred years ago. Or even 30 years ago. The government pays farmers to grow the hybrid and genetically modified grains of today (drives me crazy!) which have exponentially higher amounts of anti-nutrient proteins, such as gluten (we'll dig deeper into this later). Not to mention, most are sprayed with Roundup and other poisons.

"But humans are living longer than ever, and grains must be a big part of that," you might assume. Actually, in any part of the world, whenever grain-based diets were first adopted as a staple food replacing foraged foods, negative consequences resulted, including: a reduction in stature (average height shrunk by six inches), increase in infant mortality (more kids died), shorter lifespan, increase in osteomalacia and other bone mineral diseases, and an increase in cavities and enamel defects. A decrease in brain size was also seen!

People often like to bring up the fact that, on average, people today live longer than our ancestors did, and somehow, they think our current diet is the reason for that. Our ancestors lived to about 42 years old, but that number is deceiving. Giving birth in the woods is dangerous. Could you imagine? Not only giving birth outside but then living outside every minute of every day. Because of this, infant mortality was high. Add to that the absence of emergency rooms where doctors could save you after a trauma. Hunting large game with a spear would also be dangerous. Still, many of our ancestors lived to an old age. When a bunch of people live into their eighties and a bunch of others are dying very young, the average age is 42. Everyone wasn't simply falling apart in their thirties and then dying up until grains increased humans' lifespans.

When humans first moved to crowded cities with high-grain diets, life expectancy actually dropped to about 20! In every instance, big jumps in life expectancy were not because old people are getting older, they happened because less children were dying.

But whole grains have fiber and we need lots of fiber, right? It is true humans need to eat more fiber, but there are two types of fiber. The fiber in grains is very different from the fiber in fruits and vegetables. The fruit and veggie fiber is what humans really need. I'm sure you're aware that fiber helps with healthy poops. Fiber is a great pipe cleaner.

What Is Fiber?

Fiber is just a carbohydrate. It's a carbohydrate that's in a form your body can't digest, that can't be broken down. This is extremely important. There are two kinds of fiber: water-*soluble* fiber, which is the great fiber that we really need, and water-*insoluble* fiber which is also good. But the best source of soluble fiber, by far, is fruits and vegetables.

There are a number of reasons why water-soluble fiber is so necessary. One reason is because it fills you up and slows the breakdown of carbs and this slows the absorption of sugar. When you eat low-fiber carbs, you get a sugar rush, then a crash, and then a short time after eating, you're starving for something sugary again! It's a vicious cycle you are going to break!

Another extremely important feature of soluble fiber is it feeds the healthy bacteria in your gut. Inside your digestive system live—or should live—two to five pounds of good healthy bacteria. Like any living organisms, they need to eat to survive and they feed on water-soluble fiber. Many people don't eat enough fruits and vegetables which means these healthy bacteria can't survive. When healthy, these bacteria produce vitamins, have a massive role in immune function, are extremely important for weight loss, affect our mood, and do many more things I'll cover in detail later.

When a mother is breastfeeding, she produces sugars that are of no use to the baby besides their one and only purpose, to feed the bacteria in the baby's gut. I'd say that's a good indicator of how important these bacteria are! The word *prebiotic* really just means soluble fiber which is healthy bacteria food.

I will concede that some fiber is better than no fiber, but fruit and veggie fiber is far superior to the fiber found in grains. "But humans need carbohydrates, and grains are a great way to get them!" you may protest. Actually, there is NO human requirement for carbohydrates. The truth is, you don't need to eat carbs at all. There is no such thing as an "essential carb". We DO require fats and proteins, but the truth is, humans can not only survive, but possibly thrive, on a carb-free diet.

Your body can create sugar from fats and proteins. I wouldn't recommend going carb-free though—we are going to go *healthy* carb!

I am not saying that all carbs are bad. What's most important is the TYPE of carbs you eat. When you think carbs, what do you think of? I'm going to guess you're thinking, *breads, pastas, muffins, bagels, waffles, etc.*, because that's what you've been marketed to view as carbs. Guess what: **Every fruit and every vegetable is a carbohydrate!** Here is the simple truth: I'm going to show you how to get all of the carbs you need from fruits, vegetables and tubers. You will get all the carbs you need, far more vitamins and minerals, loads of soluble fiber, and you're going to love it! It's almost impossible to overeat fruits and veggies. They're just so good for you, and they're loaded with great fiber that will fill you up and prevent overeating.

There isn't a single nutrient in grains that you won't get more of by following the eating plan I will provide!

Fruit juice should be viewed differently! I would NOT call juice healthy. If I gave you six large apples and challenged you to eat all six, it would be very tough. That's because apples are full of fiber and would fill you up, making it very difficult to eat six whole apples in one sitting. But if I squeezed the juice—the sugar water—out of six apples, could you drink that? Absolutely, it'd be easy. Fruit juice is basically just sugar water. It's not the health food that it's been marketed as.

You may be thinking orange juice is a great source of vitamin C. This is the result of brilliant marketing by orange growers. Each year, copious amounts of oranges ripened and while many were sold, many would also rot.

These growers used those extra oranges to produce orange juice, advertised as a great source of vitamin C, and created a huge market. Brilliant business! Broccoli, Brussels sprouts, strawberries, chili peppers, and many other fruits and veggies have more vitamin C than orange juice does!

Is it possible to eat too much fruit? Yes, it is possible if you really tried to. However, I have yet to meet a person that is overweight and struggling because of fruit. "Dr. Czys, when I eat one apple, I eat the whole bag!" I haven't heard that yet! As long as it is WHOLE fruit and NOT fruit juice, you'll be okay.

What about dried fruit? Be very careful with this! Dried fruit is often sweetened which just means more sugar added to it. A lot of dried fruit is basically just balls of sugar, which is why they are so sweet and tasty. A client showed me a low-sugar blended coffee drink that contained three dates. Those 3 dates contained about 48 grams or 12 spoonfuls of sugar and very little fiber. Banana chips are another dried fruit people mistakenly think are healthy. Full, whole fruit is always the best option!

Again, there is absolutely NO nutritional reason to eat grains! I should add that my advice is based on eating a diet that is optimal for humans. Of course, if the option is either eat grains or starve, then eat grains. Most people reading this book are extremely wealthy relative to world standards and have the ability to choose what foods to purchase.

I must also add that **when it comes to health, "fine" is not good enough for me.**

"My kids ate pancakes most days and turned out fine." This statement is utterly repulsive to me. I don't want to feel *fine*. I don't want my kid to feel *fine*. I want to feel *great*! And I especially want my kid's health to be great. For that reason, we both eat superior food.

"Okay, but what about grains in moderation?" Moderation is acceptable if you want to feel only moderately good, have moderate health, and look moderately well. The whole idea of "moderation" is senseless when it comes to health.

Let's Dig a Little Deeper into Why You Should Be Avoiding Grains

Grains are carbs, carbs are sugars, and the ingestion of excess sugar causes your body to release a lot of insulin. Insulin is a hormone that pulls sugar from your blood and stores it. The repeated release of insulin leads to a myriad of problems, one of which is the fastest growing today: diabetes. As we talked about earlier, the number of people in this country with diabetes is staggering.

A slice of whole wheat bread produces a greater insulin response than a chocolate bar! (Note: This doesn't mean you should eat more chocolate bars.) And what do most diabetes "diet experts" tell diabetics to eat? More whole grains—this makes absolutely no sense!

Humans just aren't genetically equipped to digest grains. We are unable to break down anti-nutrients in grains, such as gluten and gliadin. Cows aren't either, which is why they get so fat and sick in feedlots, and why they must be fed copious amounts of antibiotics, which is one of the many reasons why you should eat grass-fed beef!

Grains are filled with these anti-nutrients to discourage us from eating them. It's their defense and survival mechanism. These anti-nutrients cause gut damage which leads to pain, leaky gut, allergies, autoimmune issues, acne, rheumatoid arthritis, colitis, irritable bowel syndrome, etc.

What's really tragic is when we eat foods that cause these conditions, go to the doctor's office and are prescribed drugs to suppress the symptoms, and then are told to eat more of the foods that are causing the symptoms. It's madness.

When it comes to fruit, the survival strategy is much different. Fruit wants us to eat it and provides us with loads of vitamins, minerals, and beneficial fiber. Humans (previously) and animals walk around pooping out the seeds helping plants propagate. The seeds are dropped around the forest in a nice pile of fertilizer. A great experiment was performed involving bear poop which was planted in hundreds of pots. The result was the growth of hundreds of fruit-producing plants!

While humans have been eating grains for thousands of years, before that, humans DIDN'T eat them for MILLIONS of years. The amount of energy it took to collect, grind, and cook enough grains (grass seeds) outweighed the energy received from it. And the high-yield Roundup-ready grains we eat today are only a few decades old, if that.

Consuming grains is bad for your bones. Grains have both a low calcium/magnesium ratio and calcium/phosphorus ratio which causes an accelerated loss of Vitamin D. Vitamin D is required for proper bone growth and many other body functions I'll cover in a later chapter.

Grains also promote acidity in the body. This stimulates your body to liberate calcium from bones which, again, means weaker bones.

Grains also have a very high content of phytic acid. Phytates bind to calcium, iron, and other minerals, blocking their absorption. This is very significant. What you eat is NOT what you absorb. This is why a label can be so deceiving! I've found that many people are anemic—low in iron—not because they aren't eating enough iron but because they are eating foods that leach iron from their body.

Grains are very high in omega-6 fatty acids relative to omega-3 fatty acids, and this promotes inflammation, which is a main factor in all chronic diseases. These high omega-6 fatty acids also inhibit bone remodeling which means weaker bones.

The inflammation and damage to your gut can cause it to leak. Ideally, the lining of your digestive system only allows fully digested food to pass through. When damaged, the lining allows larger compounds to leak through and cause your immune system to attack you which leads to eczema, allergies, rheumatoid arthritis, acne, irritable bowel syndrome (IBS), Crohn's disease, etc. Think of it as poison ivy on your insides. When poison ivy gets on your skin, it damages your skin cells causing a reaction. Glutens in grains are damaging the cells of your digestive system. Once your gut is damaged and food leaks through and enters the bloodstream, it can interfere with hormonal balance, organ function, and metabolism.

Gluten, a protein only found in grains, causes damage to the cells lining your digestive tract. This disrupts the digestion and absorption of nutrients. Gluten also kills probiotics which can reduce your immunity.

You are probably seeing the term "gluten-free" on a lot more foods. Why the fuss about gluten all the sudden? People find when they cut out gluten, they feel better, look better, digest better, think better, sleep better, and so on. I still don't recommend gluten-free wheat products. There are still a lot of bad things in those products other than the gluten. Plus, the shit is expensive! Take that money and buy some fruits and veggies!

One thing you'll notice when you cut out grains, especially those containing gluten, is you'll have less aches and pains. This one is huge for me. After years of football, wrestling, and rugby my body has taken a beating. It is amazing how much my body hurts if I eat any wheat. I seriously just ache all over. How many people hurt all over and are diagnosed with fibromyalgia or chronic fatigue when the cause is probably their diet? If I followed conventional nutrition and medical advice, I'd be loaded with meds right now. Would my quality of life be better or worse?

Another thing that happens when cutting out grains is a change in facial appearance. The bloated moon face and swollen look disappears. The puffiness around the eyes goes away. You get your jaw line back!

Your head will clear, and you'll think more clearly. For most people I work with that follow the plan, they say the clear thinking and loss of brain fog is more beneficial to them than the weight loss. But when you cut out the grains, you are also going to lose body fat!

Gluten also affects your brain. When gluten is digested, gliadorphin is produced; gliadorphin is an opioid that creates the addictive nature of grains. Often people have a hard time giving up their bread, and this is why. Sometimes people experience withdrawal symptoms, such as fatigue, irritability, depression, etc. People will then try and justify why bread is good for them because they feel worse when cutting it out at first. The same thing happens when alcoholics give up booze. Just because your body craves something, doesn't mean it's good for you!

So, my question to you is why eat grains when you can get MORE of the same nutrients from other great tasting foods? Why eat grains when there are so many potential problems associated with them? NONE of which are associated with fruits and vegetables.

I would say that out of all grains, wheat is by far the worst. I would avoid wheat completely. I don't view gluten-free products as good; they are just a better bad product. In fact, white rice is basically little balls of sugar with little nutritional value. I just make extra stir fry and cut out the rice completely. You'll learn all of this in the end.

What about Oatmeal?

Well, it tastes awful. The only way to make it decent is by adding sugar or fruit. Cut out the oats and just eat more fruit. Have some nuts with your fruit instead of the oatmeal. A little oatmeal once in a while isn't the end of the world, but I just can't for the life of me understand why people feel the need to eat something that tastes so bad when healthier, better tasting options are available.

Speaking of taste, grains don't actually taste good. It's the real food you put *on* the grains that tastes good. A bowl of pasta...meh. A bowl of pasta with chicken marinara on it? Awesome! Just eat more of the chicken marinara! That's the REAL food that you are craving! A taco salad is a hell of a lot better than trying to eat the same ingredients with that shell that just crumbles all over the place.

A piece of crust? Not very tasty. Dip that crust in a sauce and it tastes great. That sauce is full of herbs, fruits, and spices and will also taste great with vegetables. "Yea, but I buy sprouted grains or Ezekiel bread!" Again, that's just a better bad. Better than regular bread but not nearly as good as avoiding grains and having more veggies and fruits.

If you still want to have a grain once in a while, go with quinoa. It's a pseudo-grain, a complete protein and is gluten free. It cooks like rice, tastes better than rice, and is a better option than the others. You can dump spaghetti sauce on it and call it SpaghettiOs.

If you ever just pop into my home, you'll never find any wheat there. You may find some quinoa that we have on rare occasions and you may find some popcorn. I'm going to share with you my amazing homemade popcorn snack. It'll satisfy that salty, crunchy snack craving. I can't emphasize enough how much better my body feels since I cut grains from my diet. And how doing so has made it easier to have six-pack abs at 40 years old than when I was 20!

Let's review and really simplify it. When you think carbohydrates, I want you to think fruits, vegetables, tubers (potatoes), and squashes. White and sweet potatoes and squashes are good but if fat loss is your goal, be careful with portions.

One advantage of sweet potatoes is they're not sprayed nearly as heavily as white potatoes. Because white potatoes are very heavily sprayed, I always choose organic.

Here's a quick story about white potato harvesting. One of my patients randomly warned me against eating white potatoes. He worked on a potato farm in Antigo, WI. He said at harvest time, the workers wore full hazmat suits to protect themselves from the poison that was sprayed in the potato fields. As you know, potatoes grow underground, and their tough vine plants grow above. The poison kills the plant, turning those tough vines into dust so they don't plug up the machines that dig up the potatoes. I'm not a fan of eating foods sprayed with those types of poisons. Nor am I a fan of what these poisons can do to the environment.

Horrifying Fact: Did you know 99 percent of government food subsidies are spent on crops (corn, wheat and soy) used as the building blocks of processed foods? That's right, our tax dollars pay for the growing and selling of processed foods that make us sick and fat. Then our tax dollars, through Medicaid and Medicare, also pay for chronic diseases caused by sugar and processed foods.

The food industry spends $10 billion on marketing junk food to our kids every year (Nestle, PhD, MPH 2006). This unregulated food marketing targets not only children, but the underserved and minorities as well, pushing the industrial foods responsible for our epidemic of childhood obesity.

Organic Vs Non-Organic Foods

Let's say you have two apples with the exact same nutrient content. However, one has poison on it, and one doesn't. Which one would you prefer to eat? Which would you give to your kids?

What if you have two genetically identical chickens? One chicken is given feed full of grains sprayed with Roundup and filled with antibiotics. The other chicken is given food that has not been sprayed and is not filled with antibiotics. I'd pay a little more money for the poison-free foods.

I understand that eating 100 percent organic is very expensive. Produce that is sprayed the heaviest, including apples and any sort of berries and white potatoes, should be bought organic. Buy non-organic produce that isn't sprayed very heavily, like avocados. This is a good list to refer to and is updated by ewg.org each year.

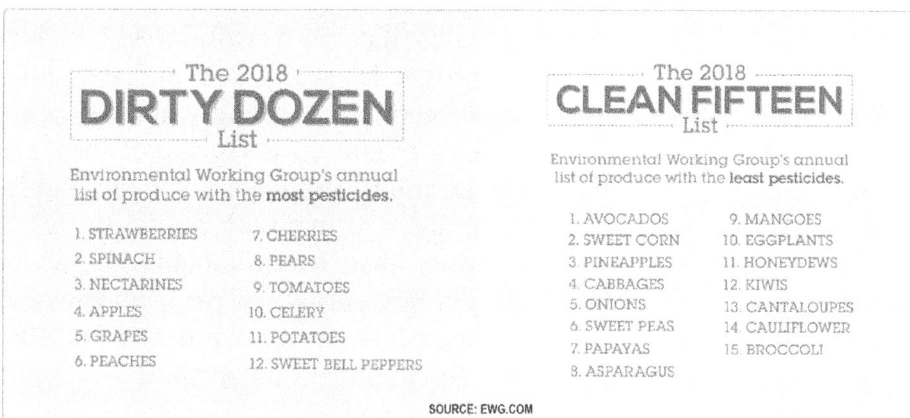

Source: Environmental Working Group

For meat products, ALWAYS buy free range and drug free!

To review, let's make carbohydrates really simple: fruits, veggies, potatoes and squashes. In the recipes and meal plan at the end of the book, I show you exactly how to easily incorporate them into your diet and make them family approved!

CHOOSING THE RIGHT FATS AND PROTEINS

"Meat is bad! Meat causes cancer!" **Nonsense!** Let me explain where these fear-mongering headlines come from. A survey is conducted in which people are asked what they eat and what health problems they have and then the survey takers try to make correlations.

The problem with this is that the people are eating disgusting conventionally raised meats (explained shortly) and they also eat more refined grains, smoke more, and exercise less, along with other unhealthy habits. Yet, "meat" is declared the bad guy. These studies also ask people what they've eaten over the past few years. Most people can't remember what they ate yesterday much less years ago. Unfortunately, most of these studies are useless because the data collection methods are so poor.

How the livestock is raised is very critical. Let's compare two genetically identical steers, identical twin brothers. One steer is locked in a barn and fed corn (or candy) that is filled with antibiotics. The corn causes the steer to gain weight and get fat really fast, and it's given antibiotics because corn often makes cattle sick and causes chronic diarrhea. Why? Because cows aren't meant to eat grains! They are meant to eat greens! For a cow (the milk producer), it's even worse. Many of the conventional cows are given grains with antibiotics AND hormones (in the USA) so they produce absurd amounts of milk. When you eat meat from these animals, you are eating the drugs in them as well. These antibiotics can kill the good bacteria in your gut, and this can also promote fat gain for you! The main reason antibiotics are put in chicken feed is to make them grow much faster.

On the flip side, poorly-fed beef's brother is out in a pasture just roaming around enjoying the days, eating grasses and forbs. Do you think the meat and nutrient profile of these two animals is even remotely similar? Absolutely not! "Meat" quality and health depend on how the animal was raised—any animal!

A fish raised in a farm and fed pellets and medications is something I would never eat. A chicken or turkey locked in a shed and fed antibiotic-filled grains is something I would never eat. A cow that is locked in a barn given antibiotics and hormones for years and years until she stops producing milk is something I would never eat. That's where your fast food beef comes from...disgusting. The meat-like substances you get from fast food joints are meat scraps from the unhealthiest animals and shaped into a nugget or patty. Please don't feed this to your kids.

If you've ever eaten eggs from chickens that are truly free ranging and eat what they are supposed to, you know how big of a difference diet makes. Free-range eggs taste so much better, are creamier, and have a much higher vitamin and mineral content.

Not only is conventionally raised meat terrible for us, the way these animals are raised and treated is wrong in my opinion. The conventional method of raising animals is also hard on the environment. A free ranging, grass-fed animal is healthier and better for the environment, and better for you!

When a beef is raised on grasses and forbs, a different fat profile is produced within the meat. It will have much higher levels of anti-inflammatory omega-3 fats. I'll cover the importance of these fats in detail in a later chapter. When herbivores like cattle eat grasses, they can digest the fiber in grass that we cannot. They take this fiber and turn it into fat and muscle that is packed full of vitamins and minerals. Meat is a wonderful source of B12, iron, and many other vitamins and minerals.

Beef raised on grains have a much higher level of a different type of fat. These fats damage humans and this produces inflammation. Again, I can't emphasize this enough: how an animal is raised determines whether or not the meat is healthy or unhealthy.

Where can you find the best meat? If you or a family member hunts, that can be an amazing source of meat. Venison, elk, moose, bear, and anything living in the wild is far superior to conventional meat in a store.

Don't make the mistake of ruining quality meat by processing it into something nasty. Some people have told me the only meat they eat is venison. But the majority of it is venison sausage which means 50 percent of it is actually conventional pig fat and preservatives.

Any processed meat is something I would avoid. I am more experienced than most in this area as I have butchered a lot of animals. All the trimmings and nasty looking stuff that I give to the dog is what gets ground up into hotdogs, bologna, nuggets, etc. Sugar, preservatives, and spices are added to that nasty stuff then it's formed into a tube or ball to make it look nice. It's disgusting.

When you select lunch meat in a store, find out if it is just a breast or ham that has been cooked and sliced. Often, it turns out to be a pile of chicken or turkey scraps ground up with additives, shaped into a ball, and *then* sliced. Again, disgusting. It's actually easy to tell the difference. The slices from the nasty ball of scraps will stay together in a perfect slice. When you slice up a solid breast, the meat will fall apart very easily.

Something I highly recommend is finding a grass-fed organic beef farmer near you. Contact the farmer and order a quarter or half of a beef and fill up a chest freezer. You're going to save money, save time, and drastically improve your health! Plus, you will be supporting the great organic farmer and benefiting the environment. They will often cut up the meat however you like it the best: more roasts, more steaks, or just all ground up for great burgers. The most important thing is to avoid conventional meat as much as possible! It's really that simple.

Making Relative Mountains out of Absolute Mole Hills

I'm going to quickly explain something extremely significant that I highly doubt your doctor understands. You may see headlines that claim, "Meat raises your chance of cancer by 50%!" HOLY CRAP! That sounds terrible, I'm going vegan.

So, where did that 50 percent come from? Let's say a study showed that in a group of 1000 people, 2 persons out of the 500 that ate the most meat developed cancer. And out of the 500 people that ate the least meat, 1 person got cancer. That's an absolute difference of 1 in 500. Not scary at all.

However, researchers are allowed to report the **relative difference** between 1 and 2...in other words, 50 percent. This strategy is applied in medication studies all the time to make meds appear more effective than they really are. I know, I know, it's hard to believe. But it is true, and it is legal!

In fact, some studies will use relative numbers to make the target product look more effective and then use absolute numbers to make the side effects look less significant.

The "meat causes cancer" headlines are always based on relative numbers to persuade people that meat is far worse than it is.

The Kind of Fat You Consume Is Far More Important Than How Much Fat

Humans have been on this planet about 2.5 million years and eating fat for 2.5 million years. Yet we've only been eating grains for a few thousand of those years and eating hybrid grains for only about 20 years.

When animals are fed the foods they're designed to eat, they produce very healthy fats in their body which is also very healthy for you. When you ingest fats from healthy fruits and nuts, those are also very good for you. An avocado, for example, is a fruit that has amazingly healthy fats. Unless you ask the American Heart Association—remember, they've been lobbied to tell you to eat a low-fat Pop Tart instead. Crazy.

I recommend keeping it simple and using three cooking oils in your home: olive oil, coconut oil and avocado oil. Make sure they are cold pressed and NOT refined. Make sure to only use the olive oil with no heat or low-heat cooking. Avocado oil is really good for high-heat cooking. I also like to use rendered deer and bear fat for cooking steaks. Again, fat from *healthy* animals is good fat!

Warning – be very careful with oil portions! An amount the size of your thumb is a good rule of thumb. The oils I recommended are healthy, but they can be considered a processed food and easy to over-consume. Let me explain. If you were to eat olives, you would be eating both olive oil AND all the fiber that's in the olive. This would limit the amount of olive oil you take in. When you process the olives and extract the oil, you lose all of that olive fruit material that would fill you up and prevent eating too much oil. If your goal is weight loss, be conscious of your oil portions!

Avoid vegetable oils as much as possible, and remember that standard vegetable oils *aren't* from vegetables, they're from grains or legumes. They're usually from Roundup-sprayed corn, canola or soy. Those oils damage your cells and that damage produces inflammation. And this damage and inflammation is the root cause of obesity, heart disease, cancer and strokes, the leading causes of death in the US.

What exactly is inflammation? Inflammation is a result—the result of cellular damage. Have you ever sprained a joint? That inflammation that sets in is a result of the damage to your joint. That short-term inflammation is actually good for you. It is an important part of the healing process. The problem arises when there is consistent damage and *consistent* inflammation.

When you eat bad fats and refined carbs—for example, a pancake and a doughnut—you're damaging your insides, and that damage produces inflammation. That damage plus inflammation is what causes heart disease and strokes and cancer, the leading killer diseases in the US. That's what makes you feel miserable, makes you fat, makes your joints hurt, drains your energy, and makes you sick, and that's why kids are getting so heavy.

Why Counting Macros Makes No Sense

A number of people teach macro plan styles of eating. What are macros? Fats, proteins, and carbs. For these diets, they come up with a macro eating ratio for you, such as 50% protein, 30% fat, and 20% carbs. It doesn't matter what you eat as long as your macro content fits the plan.

These plans are senseless for a couple of reasons. First, those ratios are based on ZERO supporting evidence. Some extremely healthy cultures around the world have drastically different macro ratios.

Second, and more importantly, the QUALITY of the macro is far more important than the quantity. Broccoli and a piece of toast with jelly are both carbs. They could both fit your macro plan. But one is far healthier for you.

Can you lose weight on a macro plan? Absolutely. You can lose weight on a Twinkie-only plan if you limit yourself to two a day. Does that equate to health? Of course not. This photo explains why listening to someone just because they has a nice physique is a bad idea.

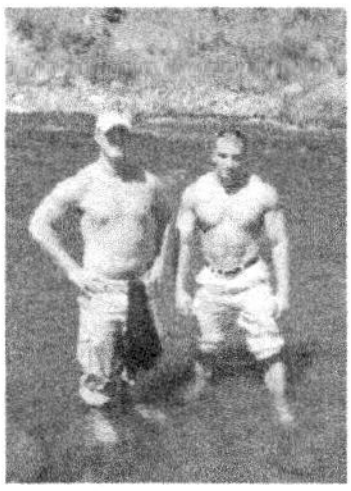

So that's me on the right at 22 years old, before filters or digital cameras. I looked healthy, I was crazy strong, I had a college degree, yet I didn't know shit about health. It's incredible to think about how little I really knew back then.

What you can't see is my chronic digestive issues, terrible stomach pain, constant sinus congestion, bad snoring, asthma and allergies diagnoses, yearly strep throat, and the four ibuprofen I took before every practice because my knees hurt so bad.

Fit DOES NOT equal healthy! At that time, I trained like crazy and all my training was based on building muscles. I could build muscle and be strong, but I was far from healthy.

You see, *what* you eat is just as, if not more, important than *how much* you eat. If you're not eating the right types of food, you cannot be healthy, period.

Macro-counting-only plans make absolutely no sense. When I see people promoting them, they remind me of the younger foolish me, and I realize they just haven't learned enough to know how foolish it is yet.

Once I figured out what to eat, all of those health issues I described earlier disappeared. And I've helped countless other people (and the people around them) by teaching them the same.

Tree Nuts

Tree nuts are great and something I eat just about every day. They're a good combination of healthy fats and protein, and they are loaded with vitamins and minerals. Ideally, the nuts you buy should be raw or dry roasted. You have to be really careful when you're buying nuts because they'll frequently be roasted with bad oils. Make sure the only ingredient on the package is the nut you are buying.

You're going to thank me for this. My top two favorite snacks: Get a banana and before each bite, add a nut to it. I think pecans are the best. It's a damn near perfect snack. The second is apple slices with almond butter. Great tasting, filling, and damn good for you. You're welcome

Warning: It's easy to get carried away with nuts! When you buy the roasted, salted amazing tasting nuts, it's easy to eat too many. There are about 900 calories in one cup of almonds! That's a lot. As with oils, I would limit your nut or nut butter intake to about the size of your thumb.

What about peanuts? **A peanut is not a nut!** A peanut is actually a legume (bean). Remember, I talked about certain oils that damage us? Peanut oil is one of them. Peanuts also often have mold on them called aflatoxin, and aflatoxin is carcinogenic (cancer promoting). The solution is really simple. Instead of peanuts, get almonds or almond butter. It tastes better and is much better for you. A lot of grocery stores have a grinder where you can just grind the almonds into a container.

Legumes (Beans) *Includes Peanuts and Soy

Are beans good for us? Conventional soy is Roundup ready, which means, if you plant a field of soybeans and spray it with Roundup, everything other than that plant dies.

Walking through a conventional soybean field is scary. Every single plant is dead except for the soybeans. Obviously that poison is terrible for the environment and I highly doubt it is safe for human consumption.

Soybean oil damages our cells and this damage promotes inflammation. There are compounds called protease inhibitors in soybeans. They inhibit your body's ability to digest protein. I would never recommend purchasing a soy protein powder supplement. This "soy is healthy" nonsense is just more marketing of super cheap US agriculture products. A fermented organic soy product like Bragg Liquid Aminos is a different story. I will use that on occasion. Don't worry, the meal guide has it all planned out for you.

What about kidney, lima, and pinto beans, etc.? If you eat like a typical American, which is terrible, and you cut back on some junk food and refined grains and add beans to your diet, it's an improvement. If you eat the way I teach in this book, adding beans would be a definite downgrade. Just eating more of my recommended foods would be better than adding beans. If you make a big pot of chili, add more venison and veggies and hold the beans. I have an amazing chili recipe for you!

I could get really technical and talk about saponins, phytates, lectins, protease inhibitors and other potential negatives in beans. I could also recommend to just eat them sparingly, if at all. Your spouse's nose will appreciate you going bean free as well!

Let's quickly summarize how simple it should be. Carbs: fruits, veggies, and tubers. Proteins and fats: any wild raised animal. Oils in your home: animal fat, coconut oil, olive oil, and avocado oil. Tree nuts instead of peanuts. You are now adding so much AMAZING food to your life!

Chapter 6: Nutrition Facts That Aren't Very Factual

The Perfect Drink - It's Almost Too Simple

Would you agree we are mammals? Perfect, we agree on that. What do all mammals drink? Water! Do they drink anything other than water and milk from their mother during infancy? No. Nothing else. What should humans be drinking? Water! When should we drink it? When we're thirsty. It's really that simple. Ideally, you only drink water and drink when you are thirsty. Clean water is the perfect human drink.

If you live in the city and the water is full of chlorine and fluoride, I would recommend getting a reverse osmosis (RO) filter. I guarantee your water will taste much better and the food you cook in that water will taste better as well. More importantly, it's good to remove that constant micro-dose of chlorine from your body. Think about this, if you get a fish tank and only put city water in the tank, the fish will die. You have to add more chemicals to neutralize the chemicals in the city water. That's not good clean water in my opinion. You want to use RO water so those fish can actually survive in it, and that's the water I would drink and give my kids.

Coffee

Fun History – Coffee was once an intensely guarded treasure. In 1727, the Brazilian government sent a very handsome Colonel Francisco to speak with a French governor about settling a dispute. His real purpose was to get some coffee seedlings. The governor refused to give him a coffee seedling, so Francisco switched to Plan B. The handsome Brazilian seduced the governor's wife! Before leaving, the captivated wife gave Francisco a flower bouquet with coffee seedlings hidden within. From these cuttings, grew the world's largest coffee empire.

I love my coffee! Drinking coffee is perfectly fine (your RO water coffee will taste better, too) as long as you don't get carried away. A pot for breakfast, a pot mid-morning, a pot for lunch, and then a pot to fall asleep at night might be a *bit* much. Coffee is also one of the products that I always buy organic and I recommend you do the same.

You will also get in trouble if you have a habit of buying those sugary flavored coffee drinks or adding trans-fat filled creamers to your coffee. I had a really hard time finding a healthy, great-tasting flavoring to add to my coffee, so I created one. The product is called Enrich and combines over 40 different fruit and veggie powders with stevia and cocoa for a phenomenal chocolate/caramel flavor.

By accident, I discovered that Enrich also makes the best chocolate smoothies and guilt-free chocolate ice cream. Kids absolutely love Enrich with almond milk for a great chocolate milk drink. You can check it out and find many recipes for free at https://drczys.com/product/enrich/.

Sweeteners

Do you have a sweet tooth? So does everyone else! Hunter gatherers all over the world have gone looking for beehives and were willing to be stung countless times just for a taste of pure sugar: honey! These days, you can go to the store and get a five-pound bag of sugar for a dollar. It's far too easy to come by.

By this point, you know adding extra sugar to anything is a bad idea. One mistake I commonly see people make is using honey or dates instead of sugar. They are both almost 100 percent sugar! It's only very slightly better than adding regular sugar.

Another mistake is thinking coconut sugar or apple sugar is somehow better than cane sugar. It's still just sugar! When you pull the sugar from a coconut and throw everything else away, you just have sugar, just like taking sugar from a sugar cane.

The biggest mistake is using artificial sweeteners like Splenda or aspartame. Remember the trans-fats discussed earlier in the book that have killed hundreds of thousands of people? Those are artificial fats. Just like artificial fats, I would highly recommend avoiding artificial sugars. When it comes to food, going against nature has ALWAYS failed! Evidence continues to mount showing the negative effects of artificial sweeteners.

The sweetener I recommend is Stevia. Stevia is a plant that is very sweet and much stronger than sugar. A tiny amount goes a very long way. Stevia is the sweetening secret to the Enrich powdered drink I mentioned above.

To satisfy my sweet tooth, I always turn to whole fruits. I receive just as much sweetness pleasure from an apple or banana as someone else gets from a soda or brownie. In fact, I find the sweet junk foods too sweet and can't eat them. You will get there too! The transition is tough but soon the sweet treats you once enjoyed will lose their appeal.

Juiced Up

Juicing can either be an effective *or* a bad option. It's great if you juice a lot of veggies with your fruit. It's bad news if you juice a bunch of fruit and only have a big glass of sugar water. Fruit juice is not a health drink as it is basically just Kool-Aid, or sugar water. And speaking of sugary drinks, the average American drinks 44 gallons of soda per year!

Let me ask you this. How is soda any better than a cigarette?

Cigarettes = Zero health benefit

Soda = Zero health benefit

Consistent smoking promotes cell damage, premature aging, cancers, and increased healthcare costs.

Consistent soda consumption promotes cell damage, premature aging, tooth decay, obesity, diabetes, cancers, heart disease, strokes, arthritis and more (the leading causes of death in the US).

Yet it's commonplace for kids to drink soda; it's inexplicable. Create the habit of drinking water! If you have city water, a reverse osmosis filter is a great investment.

What Kind of Alcohol Can You Drink?

In Wisconsin, alcohol is a huge problem! Here, there is a widespread drinking culture and what people casually drink here would be considered alcoholism pretty much anywhere else.

Typically, your body is burning sugar and fat for fuel. When you drink alcohol, that becomes the primary food your body wants to burn up and get rid of. Instead of burning sugar and fat, your body is now storing it. It's no secret that people put on unhealthy weight when they drink more. The drinking often leads to poor food choices to compound the problem as well.

If I were to recommend any alcohol, it would be potato vodka or tequila along with something that's not loaded with sugar. Wine is just sugar water with alcohol. It's been brilliantly marketed to even be considered healthy. The "studies" that claim this are so poorly designed and so flawed they are useless. However, they can lead to clever story headlines. I'm not going to ask you to cut out alcohol completely. However, you must be honest with yourself. If you want to cut some bad weight, you may need to seriously look at the alcohol habit.

Got Milk? The Facts That Changed This Dairy Farmer's Mind

Coming from a guy who was raised on a dairy farm in Wisconsin, this chapter just may get me lynched. I'm going to tell you a little story and then share the science. It's up to you to decide what's right for you and your family.

All through school, gas and stomach pain was a common issue for me. I didn't think much of it really as I thought I was just a gassy person. I remember sitting at the state wrestling tournament waiting for my next match in so much pain I almost asked to be taken to the hospital. It wasn't uncommon for me to fold over in pain, but that day was one of the really bad ones.

Snoring was a big issue. I never said anything, but I was self-conscious about staying places because my snoring was embarrassing. Gas, snoring, stomach pain, and diarrhea was just a part of life that I had gotten used to. I even had an inhaler because I'd have trouble breathing as my sinuses were always so congested.

When I went to grad school and started learning more about how the body works, and about nutrition, genetics and evolutionary development, I was forced to question the dogma of dairy being healthy. I was and am a stubborn fool sometimes. I was taught that dairy wasn't a good option for humans and yet resisted it!

I'm from a Wisconsin dairy farm where milk is a superfood! If we don't drink it, our bones will just wither away. Those were my beliefs because that was what I was taught. "Milk, it does a body good." Or does it?

I started digging into it. Based on what I've found, I haven't had a glass of milk in well over a decade. I can't remember the last time I've had any stomach pain. I no longer snore and no longer have sinus or congestive issues. My bone density and strength are very high. Now that was just my personal story. Who really cares what my story is, right? What does the evidence say? Here is what I've found. It's up to you to decide what's best for you and your family.

We will explore the dairy debate with the following evidence: research studies and observations of nature (humans and other species)

In the end, you must decide for yourself which path to follow.

We have all been marketed to believe that dairy products are a super food. We have been taught that even if we don't like dairy, we must consume it or we won't get enough calcium, causing our bones to weaken and become brittle. We have also recently been led to believe we need to consume yogurt is a healthy way to get adequate probiotics. However, is there any research to support these claims?

"Up until about 9,000 years ago in the Middle East and about 7,000 years ago in northern Europe, no human being on earth consumed non-human dairy products." The only milk we consumed was from our mothers as an infant (Copley, et al. 2003).

This recent introduction of dairy into our diet could be expected to cause some problems

"Overall, about 75% of the world's population...lose their lactase enzymes after weaning." This means that 75 percent of humans are lactose intolerant. Humans stop producing the enzyme lactase, which digests lactose, at around 2-3 years of age, the time when babies are weaned off their mother's breast and should no longer be consuming milk or dairy products. Symptoms of lactose intolerance include stomach **pain, gas, bloating, and diarrhea after consumption of dairy products** (Bertron, Barnard and Mills 1999).

Think of all the wild mammalian species on the planet. Can you think of a single one that drinks milk not from its own mother as an infant? Have you heard of any animal species that is calcium deficient or has weak bones due to lack of milk consumption? If no other mammalian species on the planet requires milk after infancy, why would humans? I know, other animals don't drink coffee or beer either. If they did, would it make them healthier? Of course not.

One study found that milk and yogurt elicited a very high insulin response. The same response happens when drinking a high-sugar beverage (Hoyt, Hickey and Cordain 2007).

This means that there will be too much insulin in your blood after drinking milk just as there would be after drinking high-sugar beverages. This eventually leads to insulin resistance which increases your risk for obesity, cancer, diabetes, etc.

This response is similar whether drinking whole or low-fat milk. Think about how bad a typical morning cereal is. Most cereals are very high in sugar which causes an insulin spike. Bathe that in milk which also causes insulin to spike, along with a glass of orange juice, and you have a terrible way to start the day. This is followed by a mid-morning sugar crash and starving for more sugars.

The milk mustache was the biggest selling feature of the "milk is a great source of calcium for strong bones" campaign. Calcium supplements and the consumption of dairy products are commonly recommended to prevent osteoporosis and fractures. However, **research does not support these claims.**

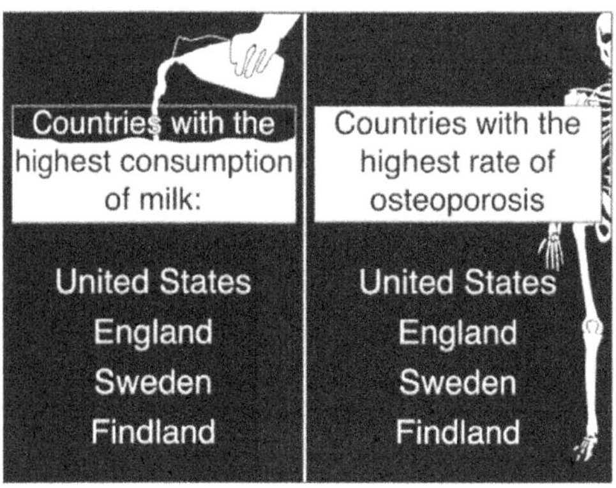

"Dietary calcium intake is assumed important in the prevention and treatment of osteoporosis. However, people in countries with high calcium intake from dairy products have a high incidence of hip fracture" (Cho, Cederholm and Lökk 2008).

"Our meta-analysis of RCTs [randomized controlled trials], which included data largely from postmenopausal women, yielded a neutral effect of calcium supplementation as compared to placebo and suggested a **significantly (64%) greater risk of hip fractures with calcium supplementation...**In summary, our results do not support an overall beneficial effect of greater calcium intake on hip fracture risk" (Bischoff-Ferrari, et al. 2007).

"The 1994 NIH Consensus Statement on Optimal Calcium Intake held that individuals who are sensitive to milk products or who avoid them for other reasons can obtain calcium from other sources" (Bertron, Barnard and Mills 1999).

Other calcium sources would include green leafy vegetables like spinach, arugula, broccoli, kale, and collards

Folks, this is where we need to be getting our calcium from! The key to healthy, strong bones is lots of green veggies, vitamin D, and resistance training! Think about this. One of the biggest problems with space travel is bone loss in the astronauts. Is this because there isn't enough milk or calcium in space? Without question, one of the biggest causes of weak bones is the lack of resistance exercise.

Various studies have associated dairy consumption with Type 1 Diabetes, especially when exposed in the first months of life. These studies suggest that the early exposure to complex unnatural cow milk proteins may be a risk factor for beta cell autoimmunity. What this means is your body attacks the beta cells of the pancreas. These beta cells produce insulin and if destroyed, Type 1 diabetes is the result (Åkerblom, Knip and Virtanen 2010).

Dairy products have frequently been implicated in the cause of rheumatoid arthritis (RA). Case studies have shown RA symptoms improve with the elimination of dairy and the symptoms markedly worsened with re-introduction of dairy products. **Milk is very pro-inflammatory;** it is not surprising that avoiding dairy is helpful for anyone suffering from an inflammatory condition such as fibromyalgia, RA, chronic pain, or any "-itis" condition (Cordain, et al. 2007).

"Studies have repeatedly shown a strong correlation between cow's milk consumption and multiple sclerosis. ... Cow's milk also appears to have adverse effects in other auto-immune diseases, such as Crohn's disease, Sjögren's syndrome, IgA nephropathy, and even Celiac Disease" (Atlas 2017).

Cow's milk is designed for the rapid growth of baby cows (calves). It is very rich in certain fats, proteins, vitamins, minerals, and HORMONES that allow a calf to grow at a very rapid pace. Conventional cow's milk may also include other chemicals, such as growth hormones, antibiotics, synthetic vitamins, etc.

The European Union banned the use of Bovine Growth Hormone (BGH) but it is legal in all 50 US states and there is NO law requiring labeling of its use.

The use of BGH has been shown to increase mastitis (infection of the udders) in cows. What does this mean for you? Mastitis is from bacteria which causes infection or pus which is in the milk you drink. The pus is never filtered out. It is just pasteurized—cooked—**so, instead of live pus in your milk, you get dead pus.** YUMMY.

Cow's milk, as well as human milk, contains insulin. Cow's insulin is different from human insulin and it is common in children who consume cow's milk or formulas containing cow's milk do develop immunity to cow's insulin. This has also been linked to an increased risk of type 1 diabetes (Paronen, et al. 2000).

Cow's milk consumption is associated with a higher blood IGF-1 (insulin-like growth factor) concentration in both children and adults. High blood levels of IGF-1 have been linked to an increased risk of cancer (Ma, et al. 2001).

"Several studies provide evidence that higher circulating levels of IGF-1 and/or lower levels of the principal IGF binding protein, IGFBP-3, are associated with **increased risk of prostate cancer, colon cancer, lung cancer, and premenopausal breast cancer**" (Holmes, et al. 2002).

The major sources of animal-derived estrogens in the human diet are believed to be milk and dairy products, which presumably account for 70-80% of the total estrogens consumed. "The relatively high levels of catechol estrogens detected in milk products support the theory that milk consumption is a source of EM [estrogen metabolites] and their ingestion may have a dietary influence on cancer risk" (Farlow, Xu and Veenstra 2009).

Betacellulin is a protein (growth factor) found in dairy products. Betacellulin binds to a human gut receptor called the epidermal growth factor receptor that is massively over-expressed in many human cancers. Chronic milk consumption may lead to cancer.

Casein is the main protein found in cow's milk and is **concentrated in cheese.** Casein has been shown to break down to produce casomorphin, an opioid that appears to act primarily as a histamine releaser. This is why allergic responses such as congestion and mucus production are so common with milk consumption. This mucus can cause difficulty breathing, as well as snoring. **Acne is also a common result of dairy consumption.** I have seen countless patients' acne completely clear up just by cutting dairy from their diet. (Kurek, et al. 1992).

Casein is often labeled as sodium caseinate, calcium caseinate, or milk protein. The purpose of casein in foods is to enhance properties such as whipping and foaming, thickening, emulsification and texture, and to increase protein content. It is often found in protein bars, drinks, soups, ice cream, pastas, snacks and other packaged goods.

Casein has a molecular structure very similar to gluten. They both react with opiate receptors in the brain, thus mimicking the effects of opiate drugs like heroin and morphine. **No wonder it is so hard for some people to give up their cheese or bread!**

Like gluten, casein from dairy has been implicated in autism, ADHD, schizophrenia, and other psychological disorders (Millard, et al. 2008).

Although more research needs to be done, the current evidence strongly suggests cow's milk may be implicated in a variety of autoimmune diseases, certain cancers, some psychological disorders, as well as acne.

Despite being rich in calcium, the net effect of the high acid load, high level of phosphorous, high calcium magnesium ratio, and poor bio-availability, makes dairy a **very poor choice as a source of calcium.**

Naturally, a cow would eat grass which would produce calcium rich milk. Today's cattle are fed grains which doesn't produce naturally occurring calcium in milk. Milk then has to be fortified with a very poorly absorbed form of calcium. Think about that.

Supplemental calcium is added to milk and then you are told you need milk to get your calcium!

Fortunately, we live in a part of the world where we have a choice. We can choose to drink milk to get calcium and stronger bones (there is **no evidence** to support this theory). Or, we can eat fruits and veggies, meat, nuts, and eggs, drink water, and do resistance exercises—lift some weights!

You must understand this as it is so crucial. Just as you can't sit around building stronger muscles by taking protein pills or protein shakes, you can't build strong bones by sitting around taking calcium pills or drinking milk!

Wolff's law states that bones in a healthy person or animal will adapt to the loads under which they are placed. Translation: If you want strong bones, lift heavy stuff at every age!

Milk: does it really do a body good?

Many times, I've heard and read nutritionists say anyone that recommends eliminating an entire "food group" is crazy. Who established these "food groups"? It was a marketing term created by the United States Department of Agriculture in the 1950s. Do you think the goal of the USDA was to use sound research and develop the healthiest nutrition guidelines possible? Or, do you think the goal was to sell agricultural products, such as milk?

What about raw milk from grass-fed cows or goats? I would say that it is far better than conventional dairy products. Yet, unfortunately, illegal to buy from or sell in stores in most states. If you have access to it and like it and choose to drink, that's perfectly okay. The fat from raw, grass-fed milk is, by far, the healthiest component of milk.

Of any dairy products, I'll use butter or ghee on occasion. I never consume milk or yogurt. If you do choose to have butter or ghee, make sure to buy organic. This is one product I would always buy organic.

What about yogurt? I guarantee that yogurt, like soy as a health food, is a stroke of marketing genius. It's not a health food! Eating yogurt involves the dairy issues I referenced above to begin with, and then a bunch of sugar or artificial sweetener is added. Researchers analyzed more than 900 yogurt brands found in UK supermarkets and found that only 9 percent could be classed as low in sugar—containing less than 5 grams of sugar per 100 grams—while just 2 percent of children's yogurts were low in sugar. The probiotic claims about yogurt are purely for marketing, and only a few strains and a tiny amount of probiotics can be found in the yogurt. Not nearly enough to be of benefit to you. Greek yogurt? Again, more marketing nonsense. What makes Greek yogurt better? Exactly! It's just marketing! Yogurt is yet another one of those gimmicky foods that is marketed as a health food and simply isn't.

Give it six weeks. Cut out dairy for six weeks and see how you feel. After six weeks, have some conventional dairy and see how your body responds. At the six-week mark, when you add dairy back into your diet, I will be shocked if you don't have a bad reaction. My eating plan at the end will show you how easy cutting out dairy can be!

Are You Having Birthday Cake for Breakfast without Even Knowing?

Would you agree it would be a bad idea to feed your kids birthday cake for breakfast? What if you invited guests for breakfast and just gave them birthday cake? Think they'd be shocked?

So, what's a birthday cake made of? Refined grains, sugar, milk, eggs and some sugar frosting on top. What's a pancake made of? Refined grains, sugar, milk, eggs, and liquid frosting on top. What's a waffle made of? What's a muffin made of? Cereal? How many typical breakfasts are really just birthday cake in different shapes?

It's common to have some juice on the side, which is just pure sugar-water. How many kids start their day off with birthday cake and sugar-water? All they're getting is a massive amount of sugar and ZERO soluble fiber, minimal healthy fat and protein, and almost no vitamins and minerals. They are literally overfed and starving at the same time!

Here's what happens when you eat so many sugars for breakfast. You get a sugar rush then crash and by mid-morning, you're starving, and crave more sugary foods. You will subconsciously eat more throughout the day.

Fascinating studies have been conducted in which two groups of people were given 500-calorie breakfasts comprised of different foods. One group received 500 calories of grains (carbs) and the other group received a 500-calorie breakfast of healthy fats and protein. The fat and protein group subconsciously ate far less throughout the day! Just by starting your day with great tasting, healthy fats and proteins, you eat less and lose more! That's why I choose breakfasts that are so different and much better than the typical American's. Don't worry, I will show you exactly how to do it.

I'm sure you've heard the phrase, "Breakfast is the most important meal of the day." That advice comes from studies paid for by the companies that make the crappy breakfast foods most people eat! I am almost never hungry when I first wake up. My first meal is usually about three or four hours after I get up. Don't force yourself to eat if you're not hungry! If you do like to have an early breakfast, eat the way I show you. If you don't like to eat breakfast, that's perfectly fine!

I want to dispel the "Don't eat at night" myth as well. Typically, I have my biggest meal before my 8 p.m. bedtime which is still relatively early. I eat light during the day and have a big meal at night before bed. Keep in mind, **predators don't hunt on a full stomach!** When I have a big meal, it slows me down and that makes sense. When you have food in your stomach, the digestion process takes energy and pulls blood from your extremities. This is why working out after a big meal is so hard and not a good idea.

Recent research shows the benefit of eating within a "metabolic window." What this means is to keep your meals within a 10- to 12-hour period. So, if you have breakfast at 8 a.m., don't eat past 6 to 8 p.m. It gives your body a chance to do other things instead of just digesting food all day and night.

What about Intermittent Fasting?

Fasting has health benefits and can be a part of a healthy lifestyle. During a fasting state, your body is basically "pruning the tree." It is cleaning up damaged cells and repairing. Are fasting and eating within a metabolic window good tools for weight loss? I think both activities force a person to consume less food overall and consuming less food will obviously help with weight loss.

Remember that doughnut that I said was poison? Let's revisit that doughnut. It's made from refined grains, which is sugar, gluten and more bad stuff; it's deep fried in trans fats and then *more* sugar is spread on top of it. You get trans fats, sugar, more sugar, a bunch of gluten and all the other stuff in grains that is bad; how can anyone say that's anything but poison?

LET'S CELEBRATE! YOU'LL NEVER COUNT CALORIES AGAIN!

I want to explain to you why the calories listed on a label and the calories you burn during a workout are often very misleading. Calories within a meal are not the same as the calories your body utilizes or digests!

Processed foods are already "pre-digested" or partially broken down. Let's say you eat 500 calories of processed food and 500 calories of whole food. You will actually *absorb* more calories from the processed food. Same number of calories going in, but one kind packs more inches on the thighs.

Just by eating almond butter instead of whole almonds, you'll absorb more calories. The ground-up almonds are already partially broken down so your body will be able to digest it easier. Also, it takes energy to digest food. Energy comes from burning calories. Processed foods take little energy to digest because they are already partially broken down. Whole foods take more energy, or more calorie burning, to digest. Twenty to thirty percent of the calories within protein you eat are burned up by the energy it takes to digest the protein.

Less than five percent of the calories from processed carbs are burned up during the digestion process. The rest could be racing to build fat!

So, let's say you eat 1,000 (for easy math) calories of chicken meat. Two to three hundred of those calories will be burned up just by your body's digestion process. On the other hand, 1,000 calories of pasta is very easy to digest. Your body won't burn any calories from digesting the pasta and you'll absorb all 1,000 calories. Then, your body will either burn off those 1,000 calories if you exercise a lot OR store it as fat if you don't. This is very simplistic and doesn't take into account the hormonal changes that occur when you consume a plate of pasta relative to chicken. The pasta is much worse for you.

Cooking also helps the digestion process. You'll *absorb* more calories from cooked foods than from raw foods.

Calories affect our hormones differently. Consuming sugar-laden "low-fat" foods may actually make you gain fat faster. Researchers at the

University of Georgia found that when rats were fed a low-fat, high-sugar diet, "the efficiency of generating body fat [was] more than twice as high — **in other words, rats consuming low-fat [bad fat] high-sugar diets need less than half the number of calories to generate the same amount of body fat**" (Sen, et al. 2017).

One thing I have heard from many calorie counters is that sometimes they won't eat for half a day to save up and use their calories on a shake or some other junk food. And because it is within their daily calorie count, they think it's okay.

It just doesn't work that way. The sugars and processed foods have a much different effect on your fat-storing hormones. These junk foods promote fat storage in your body. Not to mention that they provide **zero** nutritional value. There is absolutely no need to worry about counting calories! Just follow my plan!

When it comes to burning calories, the number you see on your Fitbit really doesn't matter.

When you train hard, especially with an intense weightlifting workout, **your body will be burning extra calories for days because of that workout!** The few calories you burn during the workout are basically meaningless.

I don't worry one bit about the number of calories I burn during a workout. All I focus on, and what you should focus on is effort. The harder you push yourself, the better the results will be. Train hard, and train consistently.

Fitbits and other fitness trackers have been found to be wildly inaccurate. The Innovative Approaches to Diet, Exercise and Activity (IDEA) study showed that participants who wore the fitness trackers lost 50 percent less weight than those who didn't. If they are this inaccurate and people wearing them experience worse results, don't buy them! (Jakicic, et al. 2016).

The number one thing to focus on during a workout is **effort**! Too often, I've seen people in the gym just going through the motions. I think that's better than not working out at all, but it could be so much more effective. One of the main reasons I opened my own gym, Eupraxia, was the lack of effort I observed in other gyms, which drove me crazy at times. I wanted to create an atmosphere in which people are pushing hard, thus pushing me to train harder as well.

When you train hard, become stronger, and add more muscle, your furnace burns hotter (metabolism goes up), and you burn more calories all day long. Side note: Adding more muscle doesn't mean you will get all big and bulky, ladies. It means you will have stronger, denser, and sexier tone, and high-calorie-burning muscles.

A few more tips to burn more calories throughout the day:

Standing, fidgeting, and walking will help keep your furnace burning. Sitting on your ass all day punching keys, then going home and plopping on the couch to punch remote buttons will grind your metabolism to a standstill. Slow and fast metabolisms are earned.

Simple daily choices, when made consistently, such as taking the stairs or parking farther away, really add up to a lot of extra calories burned.

Just by keeping your house cooler, your body will need to burn more calories to keep you warm. You'll save money on the energy bill and lose a few pounds!

Chapter 7: I'm Going to Save You Money on Supplements!

The Only Supplements Whose Benefits Are Shown by Scientific Evidence

The word vitamin was coined about 100 years ago in 1912, originally as *vitamine* from Latin *vīta* (life) and *amine* (amino acids).

Are you currently taking vitamins or supplements? Nod your head if you are. It's okay, most people are. But do you really need them? How do you know whether you need them? And how do you know if what you are taking is actually high quality and beneficial? I will answer those questions and am probably going to save you some money!

If a tree out in your yard is kind of wilting and looking a little sickly, what's the first thing you think it needs? Water, right? Let's say you water it and it still looks kind of sickly. What do you think next? That maybe it needs more sunlight, or maybe some fertilizer? You might also wonder, what nutrient does this plant need to be healthy yet is deficient in?

Likewise, is it possible for us to not feel our best, to have symptoms, be a little bit sick, to have aches and pains because we're deficient in a nutrient that we need, just as a plant may be deficient in nutrients it needs? Absolutely!

Not long ago, scurvy killed MILLIONS of people! All those people needed to survive was a bit of vitamin C. As recent as 1917, the lead nutritionist in America, the man who discovered vitamins A and B, claimed that the cause of scurvy was constipation! Prior to the discovery of vitamin C in 1912, one of the common scurvy treatments involved rinsing patients' mouths out with urine! All they really needed was a piece of fruit loaded with vitamin C.

The reason doctors recommend that pregnant women take prenatal vitamins is because if they are deficient in folate, the baby can develop a neural tube defect. What most people don't realize is by the time a woman learns she is pregnant, it's too late to prevent this type of defect. The neural tube closes around the 28th day of pregnancy. It's important for women to be sufficient in all nutrients before, during, and after pregnancy!

Where do vitamins and minerals come from? Food! Ideally, we would receive all the nutrients our bodies' need from food. The only time you should take a supplement is if you're not getting enough of a nutrient your body requires to be healthy, and you can't get enough of it from food.

Unfortunately, there are a few nutrients that are nearly impossible to get adequate amounts of in your diet. Those are the only ones that I take on a regular basis. Before we get into specifics about them, we must go over the golden rules of supplementation.

Before You Spend Money on Any Supplement, It Must Meet ALL of These Rules:

1. It must an essential nutrient.

Essential means that you need it to survive and your body can't produce it. You have to get it from an outside source. If it's non-essential, that means your body can produce it. So, if you're getting enough of the essential nutrients, your body can produce all of the non-essential nutrients you need.

2. There must be quality research that has shown that getting enough of it through diet is very difficult or impossible.

It is not hard to get *most* of our required essential nutrients via the foods we eat. There are a few that are very hard to get.

3. There must be quality evidence showing that you're very likely deficient in that nutrient.

Let me start with an example that breaks rule number 3: Protein! Protein is in everything! I'm a 200-pound, muscular man and I never have protein powders. It is super easy to get adequate amounts of protein via diet and I don't recommend protein supplements to 99 percent of people. I'll go into more detail on protein powders in a bit.

4. There must be quality research that has shown the supplement improves health, performance and prevention of diseases, symptoms, and poor health.

In reality, you should only take supplements that have been demonstrated through ample evidence to improve health! Makes sense, right? Why would you take a supplement that isn't backed up by any evidence showing that it benefits you? Most supplements have NO evidence to support their claims.

5. The supplement must be delivered in its naturally occurring form. It must be in the exact form that exists in nature. It must NOT be a synthetic complex made in a chemical lab. When it comes to vitamins and minerals, the way they exist in nature is always best; we have never improved on nature. Many supplements are actually synthetic. They are made in a lab and have a different chemical makeup than what exists in nature but can be labelled with the same name.

Often, supplements will also contain vitamers and not vitamins. Vitamers are basically pieces of a whole vitamin. You need that whole vitamin for it to benefit you as all the pieces work together. Using vitamers is like having a big pile of tires and claiming you own a bunch of cars. One car will get you a lot further than a pile of tires. A little bit of a whole vitamin will do a lot more for you than a whole bunch of vitamers.

To make quality vitamins really easy to understand, let's talk about olive oil. Let's say you're looking at olive oil on the shelf and you have two options. To make the oil in one bottle, organic olives were picked from the tree, the oil was cold pressed out, any impurities were cleaned from the olive oil and the final product was quickly sealed it in a bottle. It is literally just olive oil squeezed from an olive, cleaned of impurities and bottled for you.

To make the oil in the other bottle, olives are taken to a factory and the oil is chemically extracted. Then the oil is biochemically altered so it's in a form that doesn't exist in nature. Then a particular part of the oil is concentrated, and the company claims it is superior. Often, other oils are added as fillers. Then it is put in a bottle and labeled as olive oil.

Which option would you choose? Which option is obviously the better one?

This is the EXACT same way you should be viewing supplements! Every supplement should be in the exact form it is found in nature and purified of any possible toxins. How do you know which ones meet this standard? I'll show you!

The Only Four Supplements I Take and Highly Recommend as They Meet All Five Rules:

- Omega-3 fats (fish oil),
- Vitamin D (which is actually a hormone, not a vitamin),
- A whole food multivitamin, and
- Probiotics (the 3-5 pounds of good bacteria that should be in your gut).

On average, all of us, kids included, are very low in omega-3 fats, vitamin D and probiotics.

I will explain each one and teach you how to choose a quality product. First, I want to cover a few key points about supplementation.

WHAT SHOULD KIDS TAKE?

I truly believe these four supplements are more important for kids than adults. Think about how fast kids grow, how fast their cells replicate, and how much they need quality nutrition. My kids take the exact same supplements I do, just in smaller doses. These same supplements are for women, men, the elderly, and kids—for every human being—simply adjust the dosage based on body size.

When it comes to supplements, you have to be very wary of clever marketing. We are all human and 99.5 percent genetically identical! There isn't a single nutrient that you require that I don't and vice versa. There isn't a single nutrient that elderly people require that I don't or that kids require that I don't. We all belong to the same species, which means we all require the same nutrients, and the same rules of supplementation apply to all of us.

It doesn't make any sense to say that when you turn 50, you now need more or different supplements, or if you're a 40-year-old woman, you need something different altogether. That idea comes from marketing, NOT science or logic. We are the same species!

This applies to food as well. Think about any mammalian species, deer, for example. Have you ever seen a herd of deer in a field and watched the bucks eat one thing, the does eat another, and the older deer eat something completely different? What about dogs? Do older male dogs require nutrients that younger male or female dogs don't? Of course not. Same species, same nutrient requirements.

The beauty of the program I made for you is that it works for everyone! It is designed to maximize the health of humans—of you!

Disclaimer: Outliers, what I call "albino deer" are extremely rare but still exist. Outliers always exist and some adjustments may need to be made for them. Some people develop food allergies and also may need to make small adjustments.

My supplement recommendations vary based only on body size. Would a one-a-day multivitamin make sense for both a person who weighs 250 lb. and another who is 125 lb.? Should my 120-lb. wife be taking the same amount as 205-lb. me? My dosages are based on lean body weight.

Fish Oil: I Promise It Won't Taste Fishy!

What exactly is fish oil, and do we really need it? Certain nutrients that are classified as essential. Essential means we need these nutrients to survive and the only way to get these nutrients is by consuming them. Omega-3 fats are essential fats that humans need to consume in order to be healthy. Fatty fish and wild grass-fed meats are excellent sources of these omega-3 fats. The problem is that people rarely eat wild fish or wild grass-fed meats on a regular basis and are woefully deficient in omega-3 fats.

If you are deficient in an essential nutrient, it is not possible for you to reach your maximum health potential. A person doesn't have to be showing symptoms to be deficient in a nutrient. In fact, it is very unwise to wait until you are symptomatic before making healthier choices. A great example of this is a heart attack. The first symptom of a heart attack is usually a heart attack. It doesn't make much sense to wait for that symptom before you decide to improve your diet, exercise, lose weight and take the necessary heart-disease preventative measures.

Symptoms of omega-3 fatty acid deficiency include fatigue, WEIGHT GAIN, poor memory, dry skin, heart problems, aches and pains, joint stiffness, mood swings or depression, poor circulation, and more. Does it make sense to wait for any of those symptoms to appear before deciding to ensure you are sufficient in a required nutrient? Unfortunately, approximately 99 percent of Americans are deficient in these critical omega-3 fats, including our kids!

The best way to take in nutrients is always from whole food sources. However, most fish are so polluted that eating it on a regular basis is dangerous. Ice fishing has been good this year on the Mississippi River. My wife loves fish, but she is pregnant, and it is recommended that pregnant women not eat any of these larger fish. Everyone else is recommended to eat them only once per month. How sad is that? Can we please stop polluting our rivers?

Crazy History: The Cuyahoga River (in Ohio) was once one of the most polluted rivers in the United States evidenced by the multitude of times it has been recorded to catch fire, 13 times since 1868. The most potent blaze occurred in 1952 which caused over $1.3 million in damages and the most fatal fire happened in 1912 which caused a documented five deaths. The EPA wasn't founded until rivers started catching fire!

All fish aren't polluted but overall, it is getting harder and harder to find clean fish. The only safe way to get a sufficient amount of omega-3 fats is from QUALITY fish oil supplementation.

The absolute best way to get your omega-3 fats would be from eating pollution-free fish on a regular basis. There is a boatload of evidence showing the benefits from doing so. The fat (oil) that is in wild fish is the best source of omega-3s. The fish oil in wild fish is in the most natural, most absorbable, and most beneficial form and concentration for people. That is how we have been getting our omega-3s for about 2.5 million years. The best fish oil supplements are the ones that are produced by squeezing the oil from fish, filtering out any pollutants, keeping it fresh, and selling it in the exact form and concentration you would find in nature. Just like the olive oil example I provided earlier. Very few fish oil supplement companies actually do this.

Rule #1. If the bottle doesn't say "Natural Triglyceride Form", don't buy it

If you were to go shopping for olive oil, would you rather get olive oil that is certified organic and freshly cold pressed from the olives and bottled, or would you rather buy oil that is spoiled and biochemically altered in a lab before bottling? In comparison, the vast majority of fish oil you see on store shelves is biochemically altered fish oil (an ethyl ester) that doesn't exist in the tissues of any living creature on the planet. In fish, all omega-3 fats are in a triglyceride molecular form. That is the form that is the most natural, most absorbable, and most beneficial to us.

Rule #2. If you get fish burps from it, throw it away!

What about the nasty fish oil burps? Fish oil is very easily oxidized, which means it spoils very quickly. If you've ever caught a fish, you know it doesn't have a nasty fishy odor. However, if you leave that fish lying out for a bit, it won't take long for it to start smelling ripe. If you bought the cheap fish oil at a Walgreens and got some nasty fish burps and fish breath from it, then you bought yourself some rancid fish oil. No wonder it was so cheap! Rancid fish oil actually damages your cells and promotes inflammation, which is the opposite effect desired. By going cheap, you literally paid to cause yourself harm. A quality, third-party-tested fish oil company will not sell rancid fish oil. Therefore, you will not get the nasty fish burps or breath. I will often let people bite my fish oil capsules to see how good they taste!

Rule #3. If DPA or other omega-3s are not listed along with EPA and DHA, do not buy it

There are different types of omega-3 fats; the most commonly recognized are EPA (eicosapentaenoic acid) and DHA (docosahexaenoic acid). There are other omega-3 acids, such as DPA (docosapentaenoic acid) as well. Most fish oil products will only have EPA and DHA in them. You will never eat a piece of fish that only has EPA and DHA. Wild fish has ALL the omega 3-fats that are important to health. Remember, consuming a nutrient the way it exists in nature is ALWAYS for the best.

Rule #4. If the product is concentrated in any way, do not buy it

The ratio of EPA/DHA is always 3/2. You will never find a high-DHA fish or a high-EPA fish swimming around. They always have both and at a 3/2 ratio of EPA/DHA with all other omega-3 fats. Fish oil companies will often concentrate one or the other purely for clever marketing, not to improve health or sufficiency.

Rule #5. Make sure you are actually buying fish oil and not fillers

A common trick I see is fish oil companies boldly noting 1,000 mg of fish oil per serving on the front of the bottle. Then, if you look at the ingredients, you will see that each serving actually includes only 300 mg of fish oil and 700 mg of soybean oil. It is so hard to trust vitamin companies when they engage in such blatantly deceptive marketing.

Rule #6. Animal-sourced omega-3 fats are much better than plant-sourced

What about plant sources of omega-3 fats? Plant-sourced omega-3 fats are in the ALA (alpha linolenic) form. The ALA form of omega-3 fats is not usable by the human body. It must be converted in the body to EPA, DHA and other omega-3s. This is a very difficult conversion for the body to handle and only about one percent is converted. It is virtually impossible to be sufficient in omega-3 fats from plant sources. When you look at the history of humans, this makes perfect sense. Humans didn't roam the wilderness looking for seeds to munch on. We were consuming fish and herbivores on a regular basis which have the ability to convert ALA to EPA/DHA/DPA and store it in their tissues. For the exact fish oil my family and I take, visit drczys.com/myproducts.

What about the studies and articles online that say fish oil doesn't actually help but eating fish does? The answer is actually very simple. The studies that showed fish oil doesn't work used ethyl ester, or tiny doses or fractioned low-quality fish oil. Of course those substances didn't work. When a poor-quality product is used in a study, you can't legitimately conclude that every type of fish oil is bad. This would be like watering a plant with polluted water and claiming water doesn't benefit plants.

Those studies always conclude by saying that "fish oil doesn't benefit health but eating fish fat does." Quality fish oil is literally fish fat that has been filtered and put in a bottle. It IS fish! How could it possibly not be of benefit when it literally is the exact same nutrient you would get from eating fish, just cleaner?

Another problem with many studies is poor design resulting in the wrong conclusion. You will find studies in which people with heart disease were given a fish oil supplement, almost always poor-quality fish oil. The people with heart disease didn't see a drastic improvement in heart disease outcomes and concluded that fish oil didn't help. Fish oil isn't going to erase years of drinking soda, eating chips, not exercising, smoking and all the poor other choices that damaged the heart in the first place!

This blanket conclusion that fish oil "does not help at all" cannot be made. If a person is deficient in an essential nutrient, then that person is not as healthy as he/she could be. It doesn't matter whether symptoms are present or not. If you are deficient in the essential nutrients from omega-3 fats and you become sufficient after supplementing, you are without question healthier. This is true with or without the presence of symptoms.

If a person is a little bit dehydrated but not yet showing any symptoms, wouldn't he/she still be healthier if fully hydrated? It would be foolish to wait until cotton mouth and muscle cramping really set in before deciding to have a drink. Just because fish oil didn't cure someone's heart disease, doesn't mean they didn't become healthier!

Innate Choice, a health and wellness company, examined a primary prevention study by D. Mozaffarian and others. "These authors looked at subjects without prevalent coronary heart disease (CHD), stroke, or heart failure. [They] studied whether or not consuming more omega-3 fatty acids increased health status and prevented illness and death. Guess what they found? 'Higher circulating individual and total omega-3 PUFA levels are associated with lower total mortality, especially CHD death, in older adults.' [To] paraphrase, the subjects who had more sufficient dietary intake of omega-3 fatty acids lived longer and had a significantly decreased chance of dying from heart disease" (The Wellness Practice Global Self Health Corp 2013).

Plenty of research exists that shows the benefits of consuming omega-3 fats:

- A study at the University of South Australia demonstrated that taking fish oil combined with moderate exercise for 12 weeks boosted weight loss. The researchers determined that the fish oil activated enzymes responsible for burning fat! (Hill, et al. 2007).
- Eating fatty fish is shown to lower blood pressure, lower cholesterol, lower neuronal inflammation, reduce depression symptoms, elevate immune response and increase BDNF or brain-derived neurotrophic factor (Ratey 2013).

A high-quality fish oil is especially important for women who are planning to become pregnant, pregnant, or are nursing. Omega-3 fats are critical components in the function of brain cells. Without them, the cells don't function very well. A fetus creates up to 8,000 new cells per second! That is amazing. If you don't get enough omega-3s, studies show the baby is at much greater risk for dyslexia, ADHD, depression, bipolar disorder, and schizophrenia.

A study conducted by Harvard showed that pregnant mothers that consumed more omega-3s had smarter babies than those who didn't. These studies can be found in a great book *Brain Rules for Baby* by developmental molecular biologist, John J. Medina (Medina 2014).

I cannot emphasize this enough: Do not take just any fish oil. The cheap fish oil from Walmart or the stuff your buddy sells as part of some multi-level marketing scheme will not help. Two things you should never be cheap about: products that can affect your health... and toilet paper (This is a side rant but that cheap, super-thin public restroom toilet paper should be banned).

Don't wait for symptoms to appear before taking action! When I've seen little kids with a huge cookie and sugary drink in their hand and asked the parents if they were concerned about all the sugar the child was eating, the usual response was, "It's ok, he/she is skinny." So, is the plan is to wait until the child is overweight before deciding not to feed them non-nutrient containing, sugar-filled foods?

It is much wiser to make healthy decisions immediately and avoid any symptoms than waiting until symptoms are present and trying to fix it then. For the specific brand of fish oil my family and I take, visit drczys.com/myproducts.

PROBIOTICS: 3-5 POUNDS OF GOOD BACTERIA IN YOUR GUT

Crazy Fact: A single-cell bacteria can multiply 280 million times in a day!

When we hear the term bacteria, we usually assume it's bad. Although the trend is changing, not too long ago, hand sanitizer was everywhere. People would carry around little bottles of it, buy antibacterial soap, fear bacteria, and try to kill it all. Sanitize, sanitize, sanitize!

What we are starting to understand is there are also a great deal of healthy bacteria. We need these bacteria to be healthy. Bacteria are everywhere...and a LOT of it. In one teaspoon of dirt, there are up to one BILLION bacteria! We have up to three to five POUNDS of living healthy bacteria (probiotics) in our digestive system. These probiotics produce vitamins, are essential for a healthy immune system, and are required for proper food digestion. A large part of human poop is actually live and dead bacteria. Recent research shows probiotics have a large influence on body weight and our psychological health.

Humans used to consume these healthy bacteria (probiotics) on a regular basis. Today, our produce is often sprayed with herbicides and pesticides, pasteurized, irradiated, and basically just too clean. We consume a tiny fraction of the probiotics we once consumed.

On top of that is the massive overuse of antibiotics. Antibiotics can and do save lives. However, antibiotics also can and do cause harm. Antibiotics kill bacteria, both good and bad. Antibiotics can kill off the healthy bacteria required for optimal health. NSAIDS (aspirin, Aleve, ibuprofen, etc.) and artificial sweeteners can also kill our healthy bacteria.

Most of us are consuming more antibiotics than we know. The vast majority of antibiotic use in the US is in livestock food. Antibiotics make animals, like chickens, gain weight much faster. **Remember the link between lack of probiotics and weight gain!** Part of the reason you are struggling to lose weight could be from improper bacteria balance in your digestive system. Another reason antibiotics are given to animals is because of the unhealthy food fed to livestock. Cattle are fed corn (sugar) to fatten them up before slaughter. Cattle really are not designed to eat large amounts of corn, so they become sick, and the corn often causes chronic diarrhea. The cattle feed is medicated with antibiotics to combat this.

So, what does this have to do with you? When you eat meat or drink the milk from animals who have ingested antibiotics, you are consuming those antibiotics. This is one reason why free-range organic foods are a much healthier option. Antibiotics in even a tiny amount can negatively affect the healthy bacteria in your digestive system.

Okay, we know we NEED a sufficient amount of healthy bacteria in our digestive system and no unhealthy bacteria; how can we make this happen?

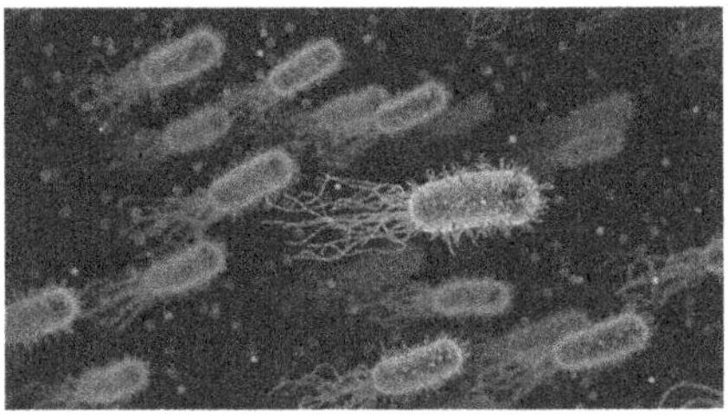

The human gut contains 100 trillion bacteria. They outnumber your own cells 10 to 1 and make up 1-3% of your body mass.

Imagine your digestive system is a garden. Vegetables represent the good bacteria (probiotics) and weeds represent bad bacteria, such as Clostridia. If you want a healthy garden, you need to plant lots of vegetables. You need to give the vegetables water, food, and sunlight to grow. If you take care of the vegetables, you will have a very healthy garden and weeds (unhealthy bacteria) will have a hard time growing. You may find a few weeds in there, but you will hardly notice. If you neglect your garden, weeds (unhealthy bacteria) will start to take over. You could spray the weeds (antibiotics) and kill off the garden (veggies included), ridding it of weeds for a while. But if you don't plant more vegetables and maintain them, the weeds will just come back and keep coming back.

The key to a healthy gut is to make sure you are planting plenty of good bacteria and feeding them to stay healthy. Continually trying to kill the bad bacteria without growing the good doesn't work. When you have a healthy gut full of healthy bacteria, the bad guys can't survive because the good bacteria drown them out. That is why some people get sick more often, stay sick longer, and never really seem to stay healthy.

Their immune system is weak, and they are prone to bad bacteria taking over.

Okay I'm in. I want to grow a healthy bacteria farm in my digestive system. How do I do it? Who knows—maybe bacteria are the more intelligent species and they just grew humans as a place to live...it's a theory I've read about.

First, we must try to avoid eating conventionally raised meats (and the antibiotics they are fed) as much as possible. We also need to realize that most of our sinus infections, colds, the flu, etc. are caused by a virus. Antibiotics should be avoided as much as possible as they do nothing against viruses. We need to avoid eating the processed foods, grains, and all the stuff you already know is bad! Those foods not only promote weight gain because of an excess of unhealthy calories, but also feed bad bacteria, which promote weight gain.

We also need to plant and maintain the garden in our digestive system: healthy bacteria. Fermented foods like sauerkraut, kimchi, kombucha, pickled beets, pickles, pickled eggs, etc. are great sources of healthy bacteria. Choose organic produce when possible. Eating veggies picked fresh from the garden and grown in healthy-bacteria-rich soil is great. Supplementation with probiotics is also a great option.

So, are all probiotic supplements the same? Not even close. Just as you need to plant different vegetables to grow a healthy and diverse vegetable garden, there are different strains of bacteria that you need in your gut to be healthy.

How Do We Know Which Bacteria Strains Are Desired and Which Strains We Should Look For in a Probiotic Supplement?

- There needs to be evidence showing the bacteria can survive the acid in our stomach and grow in our digestive system. If healthy bacteria are killed, they are useless.
- Probiotics need to be alive. A supplement needs to be third-party tested proving there are living organisms in the capsules. This is why they should be kept refrigerated to keep the little buggers alive.

- Healthy bacteria of the human gut were established long before agriculture. Bacteria grown in dairy products (yogurt) or grains (corn, wheat, soy) are not optimal strains for humans. Pasteurization kills bacteria so any bacteria in conventional dairy products will be dead anyway. Probiotics needs to be from non-dairy or non-grain sources.
- There needs to be evidence showing the strain actually improves health outcomes.

The probiotic supplement that my wife and I take, and give our baby has 50 BILLION living healthy bacteria in each capsule. They are listed as CFUs, or colony forming units. This means the bacteria can survive and reproduce in your gut, creating healthy colonies (a healthy garden). For the baby, I just pull the capsule apart and dump a little bit of powder into his milk.

There are 16 different bacteria strains, each of which is proven to survive when eaten and proven to improve health outcomes. The label will tell you exactly how many CFUs it has of each strain; this is very important. If you look at most probiotics, the label will say they used a "proprietary blend" and then list a few strains on the back. You would have no idea what is actually in there. What this likely means is that the majority of those inside are the cheapest strain to produce, and only a little bit of the other strains is included—just enough to be able to claim "multiple" on the label. DO NOT pay for them!

My wife and I each take one capsule every morning as a maintenance dose. If you have any digestive issues, gas, bloating, constipation, etc., or have recently been on an antibiotic, I would take at least one in the morning and evening for a month. I would recommend that as a therapeutic dose, eventually reducing it to one per day.

What about for kids? They are growing faster and really need proper nutrition. If anyone should be taking good supplements, it is our kids. Fish oil, vitamin D, and probiotics really should be given to every child. The probiotic is in a capsule that easily pulls apart. Just pull it apart and add some to their food or drink.

But I eat yogurt. Isn't that good enough?

Probiotics in yogurt is nothing more than clever marketing. First of all, the human body has been consuming strains of probiotics growing in vegetables since the beginning of time. NOT strains grown in dairy. Second, the number of probiotic CFUs in yogurt is so small that it's pointless, and finally, the yogurt has been pasteurized so there is a good chance the probiotics are dead.

What about Prebiotics?

Prebiotics are food *for* the bacteria. Prebiotic is just another word for water-soluble fiber. All living creatures need to eat! If you eat the foods I have taught you to eat from day one, your probiotics will get all the food *they* need. Vegetables, fruits, meats, nuts, eggs (all ideally organic), and water will feed your bacteria garden to grow to be healthy and thriving.

Would you ever consider taking poop pills? Yes, that is a reality. The poop of healthy people is being collected and put into capsules for people to ingest and restore their healthy bacteria. Personally, I think I'll just choose healthy foods and a good probiotic (grown from produce) than resort to poop pills.

But I don't really have any symptoms; should I still take a probiotic?

I don't have heart disease symptoms; do I still need to exercise? Too often, people wait until symptoms appear before improving lifestyle decisions. It's much wiser to make healthy choices and prevent symptoms from ever appearing.

Here's a quick story as an example. A previous teammate would tease me for bringing my own food to softball tournaments. Cheesy pretzels, corn dogs, and nachos with fake cheese didn't really appeal to me. Eventually, that teammate developed hemorrhoids so bad he had to stuff his underwear with toilet paper to prevent the blood from soaking through his pants. Moral of the story: Don't wait until you have symptoms to make healthier choices!

When it comes to health care, there is no glory or media attention to be gained in prevention. If a doctor teaches patients how to eat and exercise and they live their whole lives disease free, you likely won't ever hear the doctor's name. But if you have a heart attack and the emergency room doctors save you from dying or bring you back, those people become heroes.

The same is true of war. The best generals employ such great strategy, the enemy accepts defeat without a battle. You'll never know that general's name even though the battle was won and not a life was lost. If a general wins a great battle with massive casualties, however, he is often remembered as a war hero. This analogy is from the well-known book, *The Art of War*.

Congrats. If you understand this, you understand more about probiotics than most health care professionals! However, education without action is useless. Apply it!

Probiotics are essential in assisting your body with nutrient absorption, and the overall result provides you with a healthier gut which leads to health and overall vitality. Following are a few positive benefits of probiotics:

- Enhances immune system
- Prevents severe infections following abdominal surgery
- Suppresses malignant cancer cells (breast, colon, prostate, and more)
- Acts as a co-treatment with radiation therapy for cancer
- Counters and improves digestive diseases (acute and chronic diarrhea, irritable bowel syndrome, inflammatory bowel disease, non-alcoholic fatty liver disease, and colorectal cancer)
- Demonstrates cholesterol-reducing potential
- Halts and treats obesity-related metabolic diseases (type2 diabetes, cardiovascular disease, and certain cancers)
- Curbs autoimmune response (celiac disease, fibromyalgia, rheumatoid arthritis, thyroiditis, and more)
- Inhibits and improves allergies (food, dermatitis)

- Halts aging (restores acidic skin pH, alleviates oxidative stress, attenuates photo aging, improves skin barrier function, and enhances hair quality)
- Boosts brain health (cognition, memory, mood, and more) (drczys.com/myproducts)

Vitamin D: The Hormone You Don't Have Enough Of

What if a supplement that only costs PENNIES per day and has been shown to do all of these things existed?

- Improve immune system function (get sick less)
- Improve muscle function
- Improve cardiovascular function (healthy heart and circulation)
- Improve respiratory system function (healthy lungs and airways)
- Improve brain development
- Provide anti-cancer effects

Would you take it? Of course! My family and I take vitamin D every day. Let me take a couple minutes to explain to you why we take vitamin D, how much to take, and what kind of vitamin D is the best.

Vitamin D is an essential nutrient. Essential means that you need it to survive and your body cannot produce it. You must get it from an outside source. An easy analogy to explain this is sunlight for plants. A plant will die if it doesn't get any sunlight. If the plant gets minimal sunlight, it will survive, but it won't thrive as it would if it was receiving optimal amounts of the sunlight it needed and will not be very healthy. Sunlight benefits plants in countless ways. Trying to determine all the different ways sunlight helps a plant is pointless.

This is exactly how vitamin D works for you. If you are taking in the required amount of vitamin D, the numerous systems in your body that are affected by vitamin D will work properly. If you are getting some vitamin D, but not enough, you can survive but you won't be healthy. If you get zero vitamin D, you will die.

If your body does not have the optimal level of an essential vitamin, you cannot achieve optimal health. It really is that simple.

So where does vitamin D come from? Just as a plant needs the sunlight to survive, your body gets vitamin D from sunlight. When sunlight hits your skin, your body produces the hormone, vitamin D. Yes, it is actually considered more of a hormone than a vitamin, a hormone that you need to survive!

Here is the problem with that: People rarely get enough sunlight through their skin, which causes them to be deficient in vitamin D. During the winter in Wisconsin, you wake up in the dark. You sit under artificial lights all day at work. You then leave work in the dark. There is so little sun exposure, that it's not possible to produce adequate amounts of vitamin D.

Now think about this. Winter is considered "cold and flu season." It is absurd to think that there are more bacteria or viruses floating around in the winter months. Viruses and bacteria, good and bad, are around us constantly. But because days are shorter and colder, we cover up our skin and get little to no sunlight. Our vitamin D production goes down and our immunity also goes down. Vitamin D is essential for an optimally functioning immune system.

LOWER VITAMIN D LEVELS = LOWER IMMUNE FUNCTION = INCREASED SICK DAYS

Throughout the 11 years since I started my practice, I haven't taken a single sick day. I'm positive that taking vitamin D on a regular basis has played a big role in that.

Another contributor to the vitamin D deficiency epidemic is the recent trend of fear mongering to convince us that the sun will cause skin cancer and we need to live in a cave or lather ourselves in toxic sunscreens 24/7. Here's the truth: Sun is very healthy...until you burn yourself! Marketing makes us believe any amount of sunlight is bad for us. It's not. It is only bad in excess!

Experts say a person needs to get 15-30 minutes of direct sunlight per day on fully exposed arms and legs. This is just an imprecise average. People with darker skin need *more* time in the sun than fair-skinned folks; your distance from the equator makes a difference. Many factors are involved so it's hard to know exactly how much sunlight you need.

Consider skin color and human evolution. Ancestors that lived closer to the equator had darker skin. People living in northern climates or areas of less sun exposure had lighter skin. Over time, people evolved to be able to absorb sunlight and produce vitamin D more efficiently. People with darker skin need more time in the sun to produce adequate vitamin D levels. Dark-skinned people living in northern, less sunny climates rarely have sufficient vitamin D levels. What is known for sure is that the vast majority of people don't get enough sunlight and are deficient in this essential nutrient.

Now for the great news. Vitamin D supplementation is a very effective and a very inexpensive way to boost your vitamin D levels to optimum. There are two kinds of Vitamin D available: Vitamin D2 (ergocalciferol) and Vitamin D3 (cholcalciferol). Only buy Vitamin D3! It is the naturally occurring form, the most absorbable and most beneficial. Notice "chol" in cholcalciferol; CHOLesterol is also a hormone. Sunlight basically turns cholesterol *into* cholcalciferol (vitamin D). Your body is so amazing. It works perfectly if we just give it the right pieces!

I recommend about 5,000 IUs of vitamin D per day for adults and 35 IUs per pound per day for kids. When it comes to vitamin D, it is just about impossible to take enough to cause harm. I don't ever worry about that. An analogy I once heard likens living in America today while worrying about vitamin D toxicity to dying of thirst in the desert while worrying about drowning.

If you go to the hospital and have your vitamin D levels checked, the hospital will write you a vitamin D prescription (often D2, the bad form) at 50,000 IUs once per week. I have no idea why that is. Taking some every day makes a lot more sense than taking one massive amount once a week. Maybe that large of a dose is necessary to justify a prescription.

Whenever you take any vitamin, it is very important that the vitamin is actually absorbed into your body. A vitamin is absolutely useless if it just ends up in the toilet. Vitamin D is fat soluble and thus best absorbed when taken with a fat. That is why the vitamin D we take is in two very healthy fats, olive oil and flax seed oil.

I offer two options when it comes to vitamin D. I have a liquid version for kids and small perles for adults. Each perle contains 5,000 IUs of vitamin D3 in flax seed oil. This is the best form of vitamin D in a healthy omega-3 fat to ensure maximal absorption. The only better option would be to get adequate amounts of sunlight on a regular basis.

For kids not old enough to swallow pills, I offer vitamin D in certified organic olive oil, in a little glass bottle with a dropper. You can just put a couple drops in their food or directly in their mouth. The dropper is a great way to control the dosage as well as eliminate the need for pill swallowing (drczys.com/myproducts).

It's Time to Stop Paying for High-Protein Pee

"What kind of protein should I take?" "What kind of protein shakes do you drink?" I am asked these questions all the time and my answer is often surprising. I do not drink protein shakes and I do not think the vast majority of people need to take them either.

Like you, I see the marketing everywhere: High protein shakes, high protein bars, protein this and protein that. Do we really need to drink protein shakes or is this just a clever marketing ploy to make sales? Hell, I could make a lot of money selling protein. People are always asking for it. But I won't do it and here's why.

Proteins are made of building blocks called amino acids. There are 20 amino acids and depending on how they are linked together, different proteins are created. Imagine you have billions of Legos in 20 different colors; each color is a different amino acid. You can build trillions of different structures with all of the Legos. Similarly, the different amounts and combinations of various amino acids are what make up different proteins.

Of the 20 amino acids, 9 of them are essential. What that means is you need them to survive and the only way to get those 9 is through diet. Your body can create the other 11 as long as you have the 9 essential amino acids.

A complete protein contains all nine essential amino acids. An egg or piece of meat are both complete proteins. When you eat complete proteins, your body digests it, or breaks it down, into individual amino acids. Your body then rearranges those amino acids to build the proteins that make you. Your genes are the recipes for the different cells that make up your body. The amino acids are some of the ingredients. Think about how amazing your body is. Right now, as you are read this, your body is building cells according to the recipes in your gene code from the ingredients or foods that you eat! If you aren't getting enough of any of the ingredients to build healthy cells, then you will have problems.

The only reason to drink protein shakes is if you aren't getting enough of the nine essential amino acids in your diet. As you can see in this photo of me, I'm a fairly built, 205-lb., 38-year-old dude and I drink zero protein shakes. If I'm getting enough protein to maintain a lean 205 pounds through my diet, odds are you are getting enough as well.

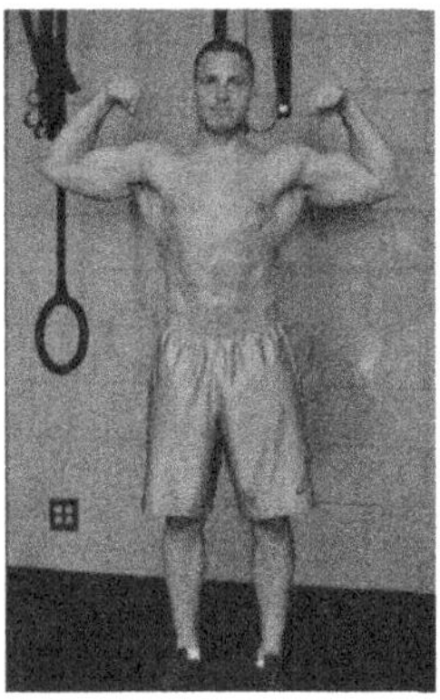

I realize that body builders and some other high-level athletes might need to supplement protein. But for you and me, the athletes of life, it's most likely a waste of money. It's just clever marketing, unless you're engaging in extreme exercise or pursuing extreme lifestyle goals, you don't need extra protein.

So how did the protein craze start? One of the waste products from the manufacturing of cheese is whey. How do companies get rid of this cheap waste product? Create a clever marketing strategy and sell it.

Tom Sanders, Professor emeritus of Nutrition and Dietetics, King's College London, stated that people were being taken in by "nutri-babble...There's been a lot of hype in gyms pushing high-protein shakes, there's also a need to get rid of a waste product from the dairy industry, which is whey protein ... It's a lot of crap, a way of selling a cheap product at a high price" (Siddique 2016).

So, what happens to the extra protein that you are paying for that your body doesn't need? You pee it out. You are literally pissing money away.

The most common protein supplement source is whey protein. Here is a bit of ironic and clever marketing for you. People often ask me if Greek yogurt is healthy. What makes Greek yogurt different from other yogurt? The whey is strained out! Greek yogurt is really just strained yogurt; the whey that people will pay extra for because they think they need it has been strained out. Both types of yogurt are hugely profitable products based on nothing more than clever marketing.

If someone tries to sell you on whey protein from grass-fed cows roaming the fields of some exotic country, that means nothing. A grass-fed diet will affect the fats in the cow. It has no impact on a whey isolate protein composition. That is nothing more than marketing.

Casein is another dairy protein often sold as a supplement. Casein has been linked to a number of diseases that I talked about in this book. Spending money on casein is an awful idea. Acne, allergies, and asthma could be caused by casein. Take the time to read that. You may be paying for a supplement that is actually hurting you.

Soy protein is another common ingredient in protein and meal replacement shakes. Why? Because it is dirt cheap. Soy protein has high levels of protease inhibitors which block your digestion of the protein you just paid for. It's also high in saponins. Moral of the story: don't waste money on soy protein.

Collagen is a popular protein of late and it's not even a complete protein. Collagen contains no tryptophan and is deficient in isoleucine, threonine, and methionine. A protein digestibility-corrected amino acid score (PDCAAS) is a method of evaluating the protein quality based on both the amino acid requirements of humans and the ability to digest it. Collagen scores a ZERO when evaluated. You won't see me spending any money on it. It's so much easier and cheaper to get the same amino acids from food.

Eggs score a 100, the highest score possible, on the PDCAAS. This brings me to my recommended dietary sources of egg protein. I eat eggs or add eggs to my smoothies every single day. If you're thinking eggs will raise cholesterol, you're wrong. Eating eggs does not raise cholesterol Eating pro-inflammatory foods like processed foods, grains, vegetable oils, sugary drinks, etc. will raise your cholesterol.

Back to eggs. Not only are eggs a great source of protein, they are also loaded with naturally occurring vitamins and minerals. Check out the nutrients listed on the next page. That is just for one egg!

Nutrients in one egg

Protein & Amino Acids			
Amounts Per Selected Serving			%DV
Protein	7.0	g	14%

Vitamins			
Amounts Per Selected Serving			%DV
Vitamin A	273	IU	5%
Vitamin C	0.0	mg	0%
Vitamin D	19.6	IU	5%
Vitamin E (Alpha Tocopherol)	0.5	mg	3%
Vitamin K	0.2	mcg	0%
Thiamin	0.0	mg	3%
Riboflavin	0.3	mg	16%
Niacin	0.0	mg	0%
Vitamin B6	0.1	mg	4%
Folate	26.3	mcg	7%
Vitamin B12	0.7	mcg	12%
Pantothenic Acid	0.8	mg	8%
Choline	141	mg	
Betaine	0.3	mg	

Minerals			
Amounts Per Selected Serving			%DV
Calcium	29.7	mg	3%
Iron	1.0	mg	6%
Magnesium	6.7	mg	2%
Phosphorus	107	mg	11%
Potassium	75.0	mg	2%
Sodium	78.4	mg	3%
Zinc	0.6	mg	4%
Copper	0.1	mg	3%
Manganese	0.0	mg	1%
Selenium	17.7	mcg	25%
Fluoride	0.6	mcg	

Protein shakes are almost always full of synthetic vitamins or vitamers and in a smaller amount then you would find in eggs; and they're more expensive!

Additionally, sugars or artificial sweeteners are often added to these shakes.

On average, people are deficient in vitamins and minerals, eat more protein then needed through diet, and spend extra money on protein but not on a good vitamin or mineral product. Clever marketing!

This is a no-brainer, really. I spend the extra money to buy local, free-range eggs. At four dollars a dozen, my six-egg breakfast still only costs two dollars! And yes, I eat six eggs pretty much every single day. The free-range eggs taste better and have more vitamins and minerals in them.

My second source of complete proteins is meat. Obviously, eating muscles gives you all the right nutrients for building muscles. "But Dr Czys, don't you know eating meat causes cancer and ruins the planet?" When you read a study headline that claims meat causes cancer, you're only getting a small part of the story. Those studies are observational studies. And the people they observe eating the most meat also smoke the most, exercise the least, eat the most sugars, etc. Yet, meat is the cause of the cancer? Give me a break. Not to mention that the meat they are eating is processed or gross conventionally-raised meats. It is far different from the free-ranging, grass-fed beef or wild game I eat and recommend you eat as a great source of protein. Meat is also a great source of vitamins, minerals, and healthy fats.

Along with meat and eggs, just about every other food you eat will have some protein in it. Even vegetarians can get adequate amounts of proteins if they combine the right plant sources.

Let's Go Over the Five Rules of Supplementation to See If Protein Qualifies

1. Is the supplement an essential nutrient complex?

Essential means that the only way you can get it is by eating it. Your body cannot produce it. Protein is made up of amino acids. Amino acids are chained together to make different proteins. There are 20 amino acids and of them, 9 are essential. The only way to get these 9 is through diet. Your body can synthesize the other 11. Yes, protein is an essential nutrient complex.

2. Does research exist showing Americans are not eating enough protein and thus need to supplement?

The fact is that on average, Americans are already consuming much more protein than they need. If we are already consuming more than enough, there is no reason to supplement it! It is EASY to get adequate amounts of protein via diet.

3. Is there a body of research that shows that getting enough is unlikely to be achieved by changing your diet?

We are already eating too much protein. It is easy to get enough protein in a reasonable diet.

4. Is there a body of research that shows that supplementing improves HEALTH, PERFORMANCE and PREVENTION?

If a supplement doesn't have research showing it works, DO NOT buy it!! A salesperson's story is not research.

Protein supplementation may be useful for elite athletes, vegetarians, and of course body builders. This comprises a very small section of the population. For the vast majority of us, supplementing protein will not improve health or performance. If we are already eating too much protein, how can protein supplementation be of benefit?

5. Is the supplement be in the most naturally occurring, most genetically compatible, purest, most beneficial form possible?

It must be a nutrient complex in the exact form that it would exist in nature, NOT a synthetic complex made in a chemical lab. Most protein shakes are chock-full of artificial sweeteners and colorings, and synthetic vitamins. There is very little about it that is naturally occurring.

Conclusion: Protein powders only passed 1 out of 5 criteria for supplementation for most people. Protein powders are focused more on marketing and profit, not improving health, performance, and prevention. I would be especially wary of any company that promotes their shake as a meal replacement. The only thing you should replace a meal with is a healthier meal! Protein can never replace the naturally occurring nutrients you find in your whole food meal.

Here's the real kicker. My fitness company, Eupraxia, currently has seven locations. It would be very easy for me to develop an inexpensive protein powder to sell in my gyms. It would be an easy source of added income. The marketing has already been done for me. I'd just have to sell it. Why don't I? Because the data shows it would be of no benefit to my members; I would just be scamming them.

Chapter 8: An Undervalued Gift You Will Never Hear Me Complain About

The Miracle Drug Does Exist

A miracle drug does exist! I absolutely can't go without it and I recommend it to every single person I work with. This drug will strengthen your entire cardiovascular system. It will make your heart and all of your arteries and blood vessels healthier and stronger. If we took all the blood vessels out of your body and connected them end to end, they'd go around the world twice. This drug makes that entire system work better.

This drug also helps you burn more fat by regulating insulin in the body. Insulin is a fat storing hormone that you shouldn't have too much of. This drug helps keep it in check. This magic drug also increases brain-derived neurotropic factor. What is BDNF? Remember learning about how drinking kills brains cells that they won't come back? Not true! BDNF helps you build and regrow brain cells. This miracle pill also reduces obesity. This miracle drug also helps you handle stress better. It elevates your stress threshold, so you can tolerate stress better and feel less anxiety. It gets better, and it really does exist!

This drug is the best mood enhancer I have ever taken. This drug also boosts your immune system, so you get sick less often. And, if you do get sick, it will be less severe and shorter in durations. This drug also makes your bones stronger and prevents osteoporosis. It is far superior to any calcium supplement.

This drug also boosts motivation, and if you take this drug every morning, you're guaranteed to get more done throughout the day, be more productive and make more money. I am dead serious when I say that. If you take this drug consistently, you will make more money. This drug also changes the connections within your brain. It literally rewires your brain to make you a happier, more active person.

Does this drug sound too good to be true? Do you know what this drug is? **It's EXERCISE!** Proper exercise does all of that and much, much more. Exercise truly is a miracle drug.

Here is a stat that just blows my mind: About 70 percent of American adults don't perform the recommended 30 minutes of moderate exercise 5 times per week. And 24 percent engage in zero physical activity. If you don't exercise, you become sick and get sicker. This is biological law.

In 2012, James Rippe, MD, stated that, "It is said that there are no magic bullets in healthcare; however, physical activity comes as close to a magic bullet as anything we have" (Zyrowski 2017).

"But I don't have time for exercise," you may claim. That is never, ever true. The truth is, you just view all the things you are currently doing in your day as more important than exercise. TV, for example. The average American is in front of a screen close to five hours per day! People waste a lot of time yet will always make time for what they value the most. Exercise is a miracle drug! Value it as one of the most important areas of your life because it is. All you need is a couple hours per week. Don't worry. I will give you a program to follow.

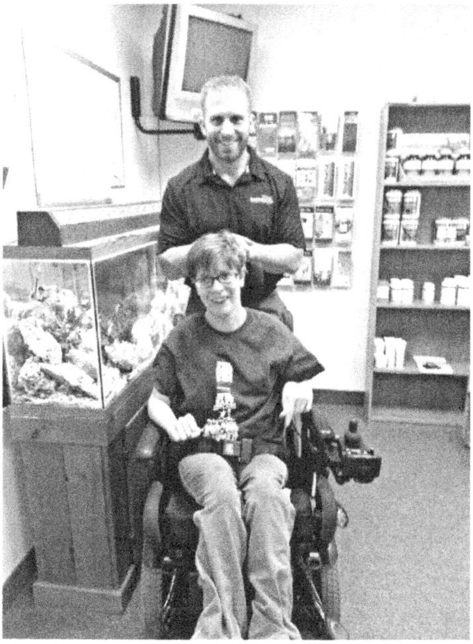

An amazing young woman, Suzi, would come to my office for massages. She was born with a brain injury and she'd been in a wheelchair her entire life. Her mind was as sharp as could be. She could see everybody jumping, running, and playing while she was a prisoner in her seat. Let me ask you this, what do you think Suzy would trade to be able to get up and do a burpee, or go for a run, or just do a push up? Exercise is an absolute blessing that we too often take for granted. To complain or think that exercise sucks and not appreciate it would be senseless.

Once the ability to exercise is taken away from you, then you'll get it, then you'll understand. Don't wait until that time comes. There will come a time in your later years when you'll say to yourself, "I wish I could still do X." So, do it now while you can because it's an absolute gift, and to see it as anything other than a gift is foolish. It's not only foolish, it's offensive. It's offensive to all the people who can't do what you can while you choose not to because you made up a bullshit excuse that you don't have the time.

Lessons Learned from Tee-Ball Players

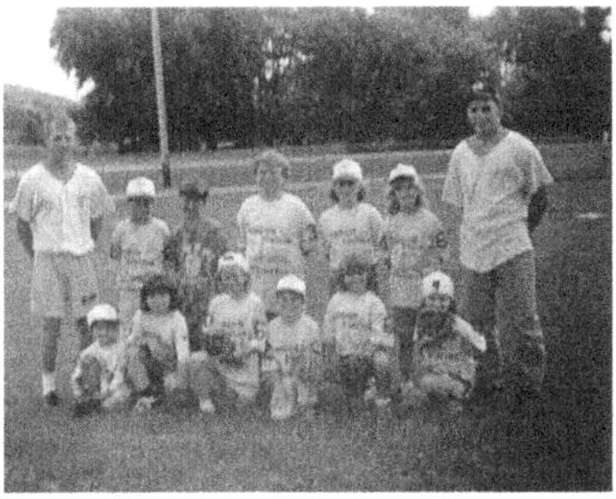

When I was in high school, I coached a summer recreation program. I'll never forget tee-ball practice which involved throwing little pop-ups to the kids to catch who had to run to the playground and back if they dropped the ball.

The kids kept dropping the ball intentionally just so they could run! Why do we turn exercise, something kids love, into a punishment? I've been guilty of it but will never make that mistake again.

"I have to go work out tomorrow." No, you don't! You GET to go work out tomorrow. Exercise is always a gift and never a punishment. This is such a powerful mindset shift that you must make. Any type of exercise should be viewed as a blessing and something to be grateful for.

On the same note, a junk food "treat" should never be considered a reward. "I had some great workouts this week so I'm going to treat (poison) myself to a big ice cream shake." That's like saying, "I really did a great job cleaning this house, so now I'm going to walk all over the carpet with dirty shoes on." Neither statement makes any sense.

What Type of Exercise Is the Best?

Any exercise that you will do consistently! And how do you stay consistent? Find a group of people to exercise with! That is one of the main reasons I created Eupraxia. My entire life, I was part of various sports teams with which we would practice (exercise) together.

The group environment made the workouts fun and I always pushed harder when working out with other people. This resulted in faster and better outcomes.

When my athletic career was over and I began working out on my own, I grew bored in a hurry! There were days when I'd actually walk into the gym, take a leak, and then walk right back out. I missed the group environment so much I decided to create a new workout center called Eupraxia. If you're wondering where the name came from, Eupraxia was a Greek goddess of wellness or wellbeing.

Find a group of people who challenge and inspire you. Spend a lot of time with them and it will change your life. One of the major reasons I love Eupraxia so much is because I always have a group of people to go train with. When you have a group of people to work out with, you will push harder, and they will hold you accountable; you can't just get up and leave mid-workout if you don't feel like doing it.

Eupraxia has been phenomenal for me in the sense that it makes working out so much more enjoyable. If you have the chance to join Eupraxia, I would highly recommend it. I may be a bit biased because I created it, but it really is that good. Eupraxia offers everything you need: the support, the nutrition help, the people, the fun, it's all there. Can you do all this on your own? You can, absolutely, and a very small percentage of people do. But if you want faster, better results, join a gym like Eupraxia and how quickly you improve will seem like magic.

If I had two options to choose from: a gym packed to the gills with every piece of working equipment I could possibly need, or just another person to work out with, I would choose the other person every single time. Having a workout buddy, or better yet, team of people to work out with is far more valuable than any piece of workout equipment you could ever find.

How Often Should I Work Out?

One to two hours of hard training and intense weight lifting per week is far more effective than four to five hours of moving at a mediocre pace on an elliptical or stationary bike. Half-assing your workout doesn't give you half-assed results, it gives you next to NO results.

This is one of the main reasons I am such of fan of group training. Training in a group pushes everyone to train harder! A little friendly competition is great. Use a little more weight than the person next to you, go a little faster or a little longer. Group training drastically improves outcomes. Again, this was why I created Eupraxia. I need that team atmosphere to push harder.

CAN YOU TALK?

Are you able to talk while you're working out? It's far more important to focus on how hard you train instead of how often. If you can talk to someone during your workout, you're not pushing hard enough!

Far too often I observe people just going through the motions of their workout. If you want results, if you want change, you have to push past your comfort zone and train hard.

I spend about two hours per week training in a gym. BUT, during that two hours, there is no messing around and I push myself hard. There is no way I'm able to talk to someone mid-workout.

If you wake up and feel a bit off, maybe extra tired or maybe a muscle or joint just doesn't feel right, take the day off. Get extra rest and go hard in your next workout.

Common Exercises You Should Never Do, Especially If You Have a Bad Back!

As you are sitting here reading this book, your torso muscles are keeping your spine upright. If I were to shut off your nerves, you would just crumble and fall to the ground. Your abdominal muscles are engaged and keeping your body vertical.

What your abs are NOT doing is flexing your chest towards your knees as when doing a sit-up or crunchy. They're actually doing the opposite. Your abs or torso musculature is preventing that forward flexion of the spine.

Sit-ups, crunches, and Russian twists are common exercises that research clearly shows are terrible for your lower back. My exercise programs show you far better ways to train the same ab muscles while improving the health of your back.

Far too many trainers will bark out "keep your back straight" then direct you to do crunches and sit-ups which puts your back in a flexed unhealthy cashew shape. It really doesn't make any sense.

The other common exercise that I'd like to see a whole lot less of is the repeated steady-state jogging on pavement. It truly is the worst exercise for burning fat for a number of reasons. It is also hard on your joints as it involves the same limited range of motion over and over again.

Visualize a person doing a squat versus jogging. During a squat, there is so much more motion in the hips, knees, and ankles. It is far better for all of your leg joints and leg muscles.

If you were to watch someone sprint versus watching them jog, you'd again see so much more motion in the joints. When you get more range of motion, you work more of the muscle. This means more of the muscle is being used to burn calories with less wear and tear on the joints!

If you enjoy jogging, by all means continue. Please mix in some deep squatting, sprinting, push-ups, pull-ups, and weighted carries. You'll be amazed at how much better your body looks and feels.

Go to drczys.com/abs to watch my video tutorials explaining this in detail. You'll also find dozens of expertly designed ab-training workouts. They will save you thousands of dollars in chiropractic bills!

Valuing Strength Results in a Toned Physique

Ladies, the word "tone" is marketing nonsense. It is really just a fitness marketing term used to sell women's products. Toning is a combination of two things; building muscle and burning fat. How do we do that? Follow my diet and exercise plan!

Start taking pride in building strength! Strong is sexy! When you take pride in strength and lift weights, something magical happens. You burn more fat every minute of every day. Here's a little insider secret: the calories burned during a workout really don't matter. The calories you burn and the hormone changes that happen *in between* workouts are what matter! Lifting weights and strength training make this happen!

Lifting weights will NOT make women big and bulky. That common misconception is preventing so many women from reaching their goals. Before I had my own gym, I'd see it all the time. Ladies lifting tiny little weights because they don't want to get huge muscles. If you're lifting weights and it's not difficult, you're wasting your time.

How do you know how much weight to use? Let's say you are going to curl a weight 12 times. If you aren't struggling to complete that twelfth curl, then you aren't using enough weight.

I will repeat this because it is so important: Women, unless you are taking steroids, lifting weights will NOT give you huge muscles! It will give you a great booty!

I think completing a legit pull-up would be a wonderful goal. This goal is a combination of two things: losing fat so you have less weight to pull and getting stronger so you can pull your weight up. That nice, muscular back and shoulders you've admired on others, that everyone would like to have? Pull-ups!

Focus on being healthy and strong, and the best version of you will shine through.

Cardio: The Most Misunderstood Word in Fitness

The term cardio comes from *kardia* which is the Greek word for heart. The cardiovascular system includes your heart and all your blood vessels. Initially, doing cardio was to improve the health of your heart and blood vessels. Rarely, I think, do people do cardio because they're concerned about making their heart healthy or think "I need to improve my heart today so I'm going to do some cardio."

A common belief is that cardio equals fat loss, but that couldn't be further from the truth!

One thing you'll notice on ellipticals or treadmills is a calorie counter and "fat burning zone." You would assume that when you're in your fat burning zone for forty minutes while doing your cardio, you're burning fat. The truth is, the number of calories burned **during** a workout is basically meaningless. When you get in a really good workout, you're still burning calories up to 48 hours after that workout. But if you just do cardio, where your heart rate is slightly elevated, you're breathing a little hard, and you're holding that steady state for 40-50 minutes, then you're burning calories **for that period of time,** but that's it.

When you do really intense burst training, or weight lifting, you'll be burning calories for up to 48 hours **AFTER** the workout.

Some studies have tested this effect involving two groups of people. One group does 40 minutes of steady state cardio, and another group does burst training for 20 minutes. The burst training group burns **three times** as much fat as the cardio group! Far less time spent, yet more fat lost.

You can also use the power of observation. Just go to a track meet or compare images of a sprinter versus a marathon runner. Which physique looks healthier? If your goal is to burn fat and have a nice athletic and muscular look, then based on research and observation, the absolute best way to do it is with burst training and weight lifting, which is how sprinters train. Getting stronger is the goal!

That is why I designed my program the way I did; I follow it myself. I do burst training and weight lifting and eat well to maintain a nice, healthy, athletic look. The extended cardio that I do (the best cardio and what I recommend) is **walking**.

Walking is phenomenal; it's not hard on your joints and it doesn't cause any of the common distance running ailments and issues, such as IT (iliotibial) band syndrome, sore ankles, sore knees, tight hamstrings, etc. I especially enjoy hiking through the hills up in the woods. For one, it's relaxing and enjoyable, plus my heart rate is up which improves my heart. When you're up in the hills and the bluffs, you're stepping over logs, walking at angles, your proprioception (sense of self-movement and body position) is improving, and you're working on balance and strength. It's just such a **GREAT** form of exercise.

I'm not saying that running is bad or that all cardio is bad. But if you're doing cardio with the goal of fat loss, you're swimming upstream. It truly is the hardest, most time-consuming way to burn fat.

One thing that happens when you go for a really long run or whenever you work out is your levels of stress hormones are elevated. Being stressed for long periods of time is very unhealthy, and it actually leads to fat storage. That's why the hardcore cardio people will often have that "skinny-fat" or soft look; it's because of the chronic elevated levels of stress hormones.

Many runners will come to me asking how to get rid of the pouch, that extra fat on their stomach. The secret? Less jogging and more burst training. And of course, following my eating plan.

Runners, if you enjoy running, keep doing it. Trust me on this, though: mix in some sprint work. Get good and warmed up then run as fast and hard as you can for 60-100 meters. Walk back to the starting point and do it again. Do that 8-10 times. It's a hell of a lot harder than it sounds and crazy good for you. Let's make that workout even better. I've met a ton of joggers who like to brag about the miles they put on each week but can't do a single push-up or pull-up. In between each sprint, drop down and knock out a set of push-ups. Those upper body muscles need work too!

When you do burst training, and work really hard, stress hormone levels rise for a very short period of time. After that, stress levels drop off, and you're actually able to handle stress better in everyday life.

With burst training and weight lifting, you burn more calories for days on end, you get stronger, you achieve the athletic look, it saves time, and it's better on your joints. Everything about it is better, except the one thing that makes burst training tough: it is HARD. When you push really hard, it's uncomfortable. I know that some people don't realize the difference between effort, and **EFFORT**. When you push really, really hard, and it feels like your heart is going to bust out of your chest, that's a good burst training workout! You'll start seeing results for the next 48 hours. And on top of that, you will be changing the hormones in your body, so you'll start burning fat instead of storing it.

If cardio was the answer to fat loss and gaining a fit, healthy look, my Eupraxia gyms would be full of ellipticals and treadmills. But I know they're not and that's why we don't have any. That's why I promote burst and strength training, and that's what we'll always do, because it has always worked, and will always work the best.

If your goal is fat loss, do burst training and strength training; do it consistently and push **hard**. Effort is very important in burst training.

Weight training, burst training, healthy eating, and cardio. Go for nice, enjoyable walks, especially in the woods on some hilly, uneven ground. That's the key to a good, healthy, fit and athletic look.

If you can, join the nearest Eupraxia gym! Just show up and follow the trainer's lead. You'll never show up and wonder what to do again. Every day, a new fat-burning and strength-building workout designed by an expert will be made for you. A trainer is always there to make sure you do the exercises correctly and make modifications for you if needed.

If one of my gyms hasn't yet been opened at a location near you, try some of the great workouts I've put together for you. Video tutorials showing you exactly how to do every single exercise and much, much more can be accessed by visiting www.drczys.com/freetrial.

The Compounding Ripple Effect That Leads to Huge Success or Tragic Failure

Suppose you drink one 20 oz. bottle of Mountain Dew per day. One bottle per day doesn't seem like much, but that one bottle of Dew has about 300 calories from sugar. Over one year, that amounts to about 109,500 calories which equates to about 30 lb. of fat! The effects from one simple habit compound into huge, unwanted results.

Small choices made consistently over time result in huge changes. And those small changes you make ripple outward to affect those around you. Let's say you start exercising on a consistent basis and become fitter. You are able to run around and play WITH your kids instead of watching them play. Your kids then start wanting to do push-ups with mom and dad, start wanting to wrestle with you, and your exercise habit has rippled outward to create a positive effect on your kids and eventually, even your grandkids.

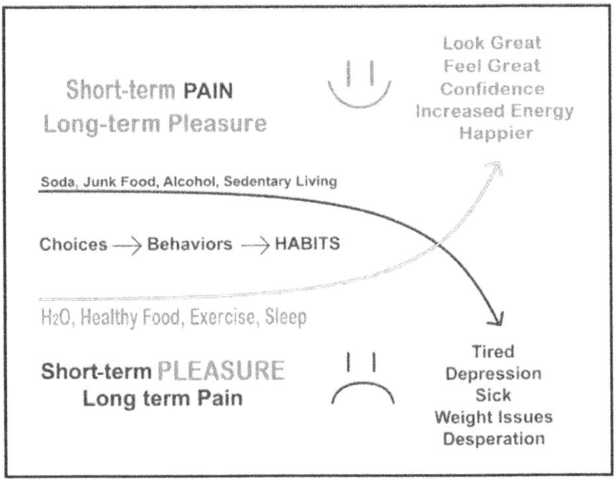

Think about how huge of an impact it would be on you and your family if you just committed to drinking only water in the house. No more sweetened drinks. You'll lose fat, your family will have less fat, your entire family will feel better and maybe the best result yet: everyone will have less cavities that need drilling!

These small daily choices repeated over time become behaviors, and these behaviors create habits. Once the habit is created, then you will start to see huge, positive changes.

Creating Habits

Here is an outline you can follow. Write down these four action statements and finish them by listing your goals for each category underneath. Creating good habits is the key. Focus on the daily choices and six weeks from now, you'll have created a new habit.

Do this exercise then stick it on your refrigerator or somewhere you and others can see it. I've included some suggestions. Improve!

BREAK THESE HABITS:

- Drinking sweetened beverages
- Consuming dairy products (see Chapter 6)
- Eating grains
- Gossiping
- Negative self-talk
- Watching more than 30 minutes of TV per day

CHOOSE THESE ACTIONS:

- Intense exercise at least three times per week
- Outdoor exercise at least two times per week
- Start your day with a checklist of things you will accomplish that day
- Say positive things about and to people
- Take recommended supplements (see Chapter 7)
- Drink only water
- Turn off cell phone and computer at 5 p.m.

INCREASE MY VALUE IN MY HOME IN THESE WAYS:

- Show more appreciation for the little things my spouse does that I take for granted.
- Once a week, do something special with my family.
- One hour a day, give my undivided attention to my family.

SHARPEN MY MIND IN THESE WAYS:

- Invest time each day to read professional materials in my field.
- Read at least 10 pages per day from a new motivational or educational book.

- Spend 30 minutes each day alone in quiet, undisturbed thinking.

I know this is important to you, otherwise you wouldn't be reading this. Make sure to follow these guidelines to benefit the most from this program.

1. If you haven't already, be sure to follow me on Facebook (DrCzysFitness). I promise I'll only post valuable info!

2. Choose how you talk to yourself. How you talk to yourself is huge! I know this might sound a little crazy but the power of this can't be overstated.

If your boss talked to you the way you talk to yourself, you'd quit! It's really tragic the way people will talk to themselves. I'm here to tell you that you are an amazing one-of-a-kind person. And it's time to start telling yourself that!

Here are a few examples of things to say, but feel free to create your own to make them more personal.

- I'm one tough S.O.B. Seriously – take pride in being tough.
- I am in complete control of my life, what I eat, what I do, how I feel.
- I'm NOT a stress eater. I can handle any stress life throws at me.
- Life is hard, but I'm tougher than anything life can throw at me.
- The "Dad-bod" is lame. I take pride in being strong.
- I can eat whatever the hell I want. I just choose to eat healthy!
- I value strength and am proud of being STRONG!
- ______________________________
- ______________________________
- ______________________________
- ______________________________
- ______________________________

A Recap of What You Should Give Up for a Healthier, More Successful You

"I find it fascinating that most people plan their vacations with better care than they plan their lives. Perhaps that is because escape is easier than change." – Jim Rohn

I have worked with thousands of people over the years looking to improve their health, their physique, their lives. Most ask me what they need to add to their lives to see success. In truth, most people will experience more success from what they give up.

1. Give up the unhealthy lifestyle.

It all starts here. Everything is better when you are healthy. You now know when you are eating foods you shouldn't: replace them. Exercise.

"Take care of your body. It's the only place you have to live." – Jim Rohn

Exercise spills over. There's something about it that makes other good habits easier. When people start habitually exercising, even as infrequently as once a week, they start changing other, unrelated patterns in their lives, often unknowingly. Typically, people who exercise start eating better and become more productive at work. They smoke less and show more patience with colleagues and family. They use their credit card less and say they feel less stressed. It's not completely clear why. But for many people, exercise is a keystone habit that triggers widespread change.

2. Give up short-term thinking.

"You cannot change your destination overnight, but you can change your direction overnight." – Jim Rohn

Successful people are always thinking long term. Quick fixes, immediate gratifications, crash diets; all need to stop. Create long-term goals and aim at daily habits that will lead to the long-term goals.

Habits shouldn't be something you do. They need to be something you are. There is a difference between working out to get in shape for a wedding and working out because that's who you are.

Short-term thinkers say it's "only" one can of soda per day. This one can is "only" 150 calories, which is "only" about 55,000 more calories in the year, which will mean "only" 15 pounds of added fat, which in "only" 4 years makes you 60 pounds heavier.

The small daily decisions create huge long-term results. Focus on the long term.

3. Give up excuses.

"Don't wish it was easier, [work to get] better. Don't wish for fewer problems, work for more skills. Don't wish for less challenges, [work] for more wisdom." – Jim Rohn

Take responsibility for everything that happens in your life, good and bad. Knowing that you are responsible for what happens next in your life is both frightening and exciting. This is the only way to succeed. Excuses limit you from growing personally, physically, and professionally.

4. Give up searching for the "magic bullet."

"Success is nothing more than a few simple disciplines, practiced every day." – Jim Rohn

Successful people know that making small, continuous improvements every day will compound over time, give them desired results, and create a ripple effect to improve the lives of people around them.

The AdvoCare 24-day challenge, Isagenix 9-day cleanse, and Herbalife 3-day pack are just a few examples of the short-term thinking magic bullets that will do nothing more than drain your wallet. Read my in-depth reviews of these products to learn how bad they truly are: drczys.com/advocare/ | drczys.com/isagenix/ | drczys.com/herbalife/

5. Give up perfection.

Beautiful women have complained to me about the tiny bit of "fat" on their belly and that their quads are a little too muscular. Or they show me a picture of a girl in a magazine and ask how to look like her. Guess what? The girl in the magazine doesn't look really like that either.

Spend more time being grateful for all your great qualities while continuing to work on the rest. Nothing is going to be perfect, no matter how hard you try.

6. Give up toxic people.

"You are the average of the five people you spend the most time with." – Jim Rohn

I am amazed by the number of people who are 40+ that go drinking every weekend. Sometimes you have to let go of certain friends to improve yourself. When you do, you will make new friends who bring you up. It's hard at first, but very much worth it in the end.

If you spend time with people more advanced than you, no matter how challenging that might be, you will be more successful.

7. Give up junk TV or TV altogether.

Television can be an amazing tool if you use it wisely. I love watching shows on nature, history, documentaries or anything educational. If you spend a lot of time watching junk TV, then just get rid of it. Use that time to interact with your family and friends. Read a book.

8. Give up saying yes to everything.

It's okay to say NO to tasks, activities, and demands from your friends, family, and colleagues if they don't support your goals. "No, I can't go drinking tonight. I'm getting up early to go hiking." It may be hard at first, but you'll find it is worth it in the long run.

9. Give up creating your own stress.

I am shocked at how many people randomly bring up how stressed they are because of Christmas. Why? You get more time off work, get to see friends and family and get a free pass to overeat.

If you don't want to travel far, then don't. If buying or even accepting gifts stresses you out, don't do it. You don't have to conform to social norms. In fact, it's almost always best to go *against* the norms.

If you are feeling stressed, ask yourself if the stress is really worth it or really that big of a deal. Whatever is causing it, is almost never worth stressing about.

10. Start with your health: Join an exercise group (like Eupraxia) to help motivate you and keep you accountable. This one step will snowball in a positive direction and help all the other steps fall into place.

Chapter 9: Creating an Environment for Guaranteed Success

When Cooking Time Is Limited, Do This

If you know you won't have the time to prepare the meal that day, than try your best to prepare it ahead of time and refrigerate or freeze it.

That's all part of developing new habits that will prevent you from grabbing what's quick and easy...junk food.

For the days that you truly run short on time and need to find something healthy in a pinch, then I have a few great suggestions for you:

1. Always have apples, bananas, and RAW nuts in the house

- An apple is a phenomenal, filling snack. Nutrients + fiber + water!
- A banana with 5 to 10 raw nuts is AMAZING! I'm serious: 5-10 nuts. DO NOT overeat nuts.

2. Meat-on-hand backup plan: Protein with veggies

- Try to keep back-up pre-cooked chicken, canned tuna, sardines, or frozen burgers on hand for emergency situations. Unprocessed lunch meat works great too.
- Pair up your protein with raw or leftover veggies. Whenever preparing veggies or meat, make an extra-large batch to keep as convenience food.
- Vegetables are NOT rabbit food. Enough with that dumb shit. Veggies make your muscles show.

Grab 'N' Go Choices

Here's your back-up plan: Just have some of these items on hand at all times. When you're in a hurry, it's easy to grab junk food; have these on hand instead!

My No.1 Grab'n'Go is an apple or banana with some nuts

Again, I always have these amazing foods at the office and in my home. Be sure to get nuts that are NOT Salted. It's not because the salt is bad, it's because it's easy to overeat salted nuts. I make a mix of my favorite nuts, so it never gets old!

HIGH-QUALITY LUNCH MEAT

I love just reaching in the fridge and grabbing a slice or two of meat when I'm in a hurry. You'll be eating a complete protein packed with vitamins and minerals. Which brand? That's hard to answer as it depends which brands are carried by stores in your area. The truth is the good stuff will be the more expensive products. But it's worth the money! I would talk to the meat department manager and learn which products are the best and just stick with those.

Meat from what animal? Any kind you like! Remember, what's important is how the animal was raised and how the meat was prepared.

HARD-BOILED OR PICKLED EGGS

Talk about a great snack! Very inexpensive, very filling and great for you! At the end of the book, directions are included to show you how I make perfect hard-boiled eggs.

That's it! I keep it that simple! I always have these healthy options around me and NEVER have bad choices around which makes it super easy.

Simple Changes You Can Make Today That Will Compound and Give You Huge Benefits

- It's time to take pride in strength. I'm so sick of whining snowflakes and people who try to make a soft, fat body cool. Being a strong, powerful person who is a good role model for their kids is cool.
- **PURGE!** You need to make your home a good environment. Get rid of EVERY temptation and all of the junk food. Throw it ALL out or donate it. You have to be honest with yourself. If it's there, you are going to eat it.

  If you have a significant other and/or kids, you do NOT need to keep separate foods for them. You have the power to make healthier choices for them, too. It would be even more amazing if you had your entire family in this together. Your healthy family will thank you in the future!

- Get rid of ALL products with hydrogenated or partially hydrogenated oils, soybean oil or high fructose corn syrup (HFCS). You will be SHOCKED at how many foods you have purchased contain one or both of these ingredients. Hydrogenated oils have been banned as of 2018. That's how bad they are! Even our government is willing to ban them! This includes nearly everything with a long "shelf-life." You'll be amazed how bare your cupboards look when you get rid of the junk.
- ONLY purchase the foods in your Grocery Shopping Guide. DO NOT succumb to any temptations while you are at the store. I try to eat something right before any trips to the grocery store to help fight off the urge to throw something random into the cart.
- Buy certified organic whenever possible. Specifically, look for organic, free-range poultry, meat, and eggs. If you're unable to buy organic, at least try to purchase antibiotic-free and hormone-free products. Buying a quarter or half beef from a local certified organic farmer is a great option. If you can get venison, that would be great! This does NOT include venison sausage that is mixed with large amounts of pork fat.

Buy local, certified organic fruits and vegetables whenever possible. Be cautious when looking for the word "organic." Organic can be written on pretty much any food label. You want to make sure it has the certified USDA Organic seal.

This is most important for fruits and veggies exposed to pesticides and sprays directly on the surface, like apples, peaches, grapes, strawberries, etc. If organic is not in your budget, that's okay! A non-organic apple is a better choice than non-organic bread, pasta, cookies or any other grain product. Check out ewg.org's "Dirty Dozen" and "Clean 15" lists in Chapter 5.

- Purchase Coconut Oil and/or Avocado Oil for high-temperature cooking and extra virgin olive oil (cold pressed) for low-temperature cooking. Do NOT buy any "refined" oils.
- TOSS out the margarine. This is another trans-fat product that was banned in 2018 but may still be found on shelves.
- When choosing your Almond or other nut butters, make sure the ONLY ingredients are NUTS! Often, they will add oils such as cottonseed oil or canola oil. Avoid those! Many grocery stores and most Food Co-ops have grinding machines you can use to make your own nut butters fresh on the spot. Peanuts are NOT nuts!! They are legumes, so avoid them whenever possible.
- Avoid ALL products with soy that is not fermented. Check your labels. Soybean oil seems to find its way into almost everything processed because it is so cheap. Soy is bad news for a number of reasons, including because it is heavily sprayed with Roundup.
- Just Say "NO" to bread, pasta and grains. PERIOD. Why? I cover this in detail in Chapter 5. I can't tell you how many guys I've met that don't eat vegetables, or "rabbit food" as they call it. It's moronic. Bread is made of grains, in other words, "mouse food." Cutting grains from my diet has produced amazing results. It may be tough at first, but it is worth it. I just wish I had done it sooner.

- Change up the table salt and buy a nice grinder. I buy pink Himalayan or Celtic salt from Amazon. Do the same with your pepper. Fresh ground pepper has an amazing flavor. If any of your dried herbs or spices no longer have a scent, then it's time to replace them. Old spices will not flavor food very well.
- Do your best to avoid added sugars. I try and avoid sweeteners completely. My sweet of choice is almost always WHOLE fruit (juice is just sugar water; avoid it). If you must add sweetener, go with **stevia**. I get liquid stevia from Amazon. Honey and maple syrup are just sugar: sugar with a little good mixed in but still sugar. **Use sparingly!**
- Avoid artificial sweeteners completely. Artificial sweeteners like sucralose and aspartame are fake sugars that have been linked to a myriad of health problems including weight gain. Remember when the government recommended fake fats (trans fats)? Not Good. The same rule applies for fake sugars.
- Add spicy seasonings to your meal (red pepper flakes, black pepper, and ginger). It can actually help you burn more calories AND has the potential to make you feel fuller, longer. Double Bonus—they taste awesome!
- To ensure that your body is effectively able to restore itself and recover from your workout and from daily stress, **get 7-9 hours of sleep per night**. You'll be shocked at how energized you feel when you start to get enough sleep on a regular basis. I can't stress enough how important sleep is for every aspect of your life! Get extra sleep on the weekend if you need it. The single best recovery tool is sleep!

  Tips for better sleep:

  - No electronics in the bedroom. Phones are off. Get the TV out of there. Ideally, you just get rid of the TV completely. Make sure your bedroom is cooler and very dark. The bedroom is for two things only: Sleepy time and sexy time!
  - Thinking and worrying doesn't fix anything. It is a skill that needs to be developed but you can do it. Learn to turn your mind off, get a good night's rest, and then when you wake up take action instead of thinking or worrying.

- Are you craving a specific food? There's a good chance you're just bored! Have a glass of water and find something to take your mind off of eating. My weekends are always full of fun activities. If I'm sitting at home all day, I eat a lot more than usual; not because I'm hungry, but because I'm just bored.
- Make sure to plan, shop, and prep your meals ahead of time. Being prepared is the key to being successful with this plan (and pretty much everything else in life). The weekly plan I have created does this for you. Once you create the habits, it becomes easy!
- Create an environment for success if you want to see change.

  Remember: if it is truly IMPORTANT to you, you will find a way to make it happen.

- Use a scale or measuring cups for portion control, if needed.

  When you start to do this regularly, you'll soon be able to do it without them, but they can be GREAT learning tools. (You'll be shocked at how small a portion really is!) Do this with your nut butters especially! It is easy to get carried away.

- Water ONLY! Sugary drinks such as soda, Kool-Aid, Gatorade, and juice, are absolutely devastating to your health. I categorize sugary drinks with cigarettes as far as damage to your body. I am dead serious when I say that. Both have ZERO health benefits, and both have MANY devastating health consequences.

  Water will also make you feel fuller. Drinking water with your meals will help you to eat less.

- If you choose to have any breakfast or sandwich meat, make SURE it is nitrate/nitrite free (no hormones or antibiotic use) for turkey, beef, pork, bacon, and breakfast sausage. Ask the deli workers for the good stuff. It will be more expensive, but it is worth it.
- Use wisdom! A secret of the wise is always thinking long term! Is the short-term pleasure that comes from the taste of pizza and soda worth the long-term extra weight, cavities, digestive issues and more? The short-term pleasure from junk food isn't worth the long-term pain of carrying extra weight.

- Alcohol. Have you ever met a person that regrets giving up alcohol? Me either. If you want to fight an uphill battle, keep drinking the beers.

  I get it. We live in a drinking culture and you may enjoy a glass of wine or beer once in a while. When it comes to alcohol, less is better. None is ideal. Instead of making plans to go out Friday night, find friends to make plans with to go hiking early or get in a great Saturday morning workout. I guarantee you'll NEVER regret that decision. "Sure, I'm giving up a glass of wine each evening, but I look forward to feeling so much better as I get healthier and more physically capable."

- Dairy. The only dairy I consume is butter on occasion and when it comes to butter, always go organic! I know we've been told that you need milk for strong bones. There is not a shred of research to support that claim.

  You won't find dairy products in any of my recipes because after doing the research, I am convinced it is best to avoid them. I cover the reasons why in Chapter 6.

- When it comes to sustainable fat loss, half-assed efforts don't produce half-assed results. They produce temporary, short-term results or no results at all.

  The weight you are going to lose is nothing compared to what you are about to gain because of it! "I feel fantastic, I sleep great, my sex drive is back, I have tons of energy, I can actually play with my kids (or grandkids) on the playground instead of just watching them, and I'm enjoying hobbies that I had given up because I didn't feel well."

The Greatest Investment You Can Make is in Yourself

The best piece of advice I can give you is to remember that if you eat something not recommended, have a poor meal, or overindulge on some sweets, you didn't ruin everything! Don't stress over it, just let it go and get right back to the good habits.

Also, don't think you have to hit the gym and burn off that meal. **Workouts are NEVER a punishment**. They are always an opportunity and giant blessing.

Can you out-train a bad diet? NEVER! It is possible for people to have a bad diet and still be fit. However, lean people still get cancers, heart disease, autoimmune disease, and many other diet-related conditions. Fit DOES NOT equal healthy.

You can invest in yourself today. Apply everything in the program. Apply the eating plan. Apply the exercise plan. Do it consistently and imagine what you'll be like one year from now. You'll be down in weight. You'll be feeling great. Your confidence will be up. Your energy will be up. You'll be buying cute new clothes. Life will be better. The people around you will be feeling better. Everything will be better.

Or you can do nothing. In one year from now, odds are you won't be the same. You'll probably be worse. You'll probably put on more weight. You'll probably have less energy. You'll probably feel worse. You'll probably have gone backwards because we never stay the same. We're either improving or regressing. So, you have two choices. You can invest in you today and one year from now have a completely different physique, body, energy levels, everything, or you can do nothing and most likely be worse.

We must all suffer from one of two pains: the pain of discipline or the pain of regret. The difference is that discipline weighs ounces while regret weighs tons.

Planning ahead is the key to dietary success. Yet, life happens. Sometimes, we have to grab a quick bite.

Some of My Favorite Go-To Snacks

- Banana with pecans, almonds, or brazil nuts – I literally just put a raw nut on top of the banana for each bite. A banana with pecans tastes amazing.
- Apples are so good, super filling and easy to carry anywhere. This is one food item I always try to buy organic as non-organic apples are heavily sprayed.
- Apple with almond butter – Crazy good but be careful. It's easy to use too much almond butter. Limit yourself to one serving the size of your thumb per apple.
- Hard-boiled egg – I think it's worth paying a little extra for the good ones. Healthy fats and proteins packed full of vitamins that keep you full for a long time.
- Ham cigar – I especially love this when I travel. I roll up a hard-boiled egg in a slice of ham. The salty ham and egg is a perfect, great-tasting combo.
- Green protein cigar – Roll a piece of beef or turkey up inside a green, like leaf lettuce, for a great high-protein, high-nutrient snack.
- Tuna pack – I used to eat these more often but the amount of mercury and other pollutants in tuna concerns me.
- Avocado – A ridiculously healthy food. Half of one is great for a snack.
- Raw veggies – Carrots, cauliflower, broccoli, radishes, etc. If you eat raw veggies as your go-to snacks, your results will be amazing.
- Sprouts roll – I discovered this by accident just because there wasn't much in the fridge once and it's amazing! Take a piece of quality turkey or ham lunchmeat, add some sprouts to it, and roll it up like a cigar. It's crunchy, filling, easy, and very refreshing.

Chapter 10: Quiz Me

I Answer Your Most Common Questions

When Should I Eat?

Here is the way I approach it: I eat when I'm hungry, and I choose healthy. It's really that simple. I know some trainers, and so-called gurus out there are going to talk about a metabolic window and eating within 30 minutes of your workout, but that advice is based on nothingness. It's just nonsense that people keep repeating.

Some will also tell you breakfast is the most important meal of the day. This advice came from studies conducted by breakfast food companies! Brilliant marketing, I must say. But it's nonsense. If you aren't hungry, don't feel like you need to force yourself to eat.

Speaking of brilliant marketing...remember that cartoon about Rocky and Bullwinkle? From the start, that cartoon was used to market unhealthy food to kids! Look at all the cartoons all over junk food packages! In my opinion, that should not be legal.

Once you really start to consistently eat healthy, you will find that you're hungry less often, and you stay full longer. And you'll find that you are never starving and wanting to eat anything. Often when you eat processed or junk foods, you crash from that sugar rush and you're soon starving again. And usually you will crave more sugary junk food.

When you start eating nutrient-dense healthy foods, you don't get that starvation feeling. You'll obviously still get hungry, but you're not completely starving and craving junk food. It's a great place to be!

How Do I Stop the Weekend Cravings?

The first thing to do is to think about your "why" that was discussed at the very beginning of the book. Why are you changing your lifestyle? Your weekend cravings are not as powerful as why you want to change!

Second, is to plan things on your weekend that are active and fun. If you're at your house bored on the weekend, many times you'll eat out of boredom, not because you're truly hungry.

How do you know if you are hungry because of boredom? What are you hungry for? Are you hungry for a specific food like ice cream or chips? Are you hungry for more meat and vegetables?

If more meat and veggies sound good, you're hungry. If you just want a specific sweet treat or junk food, you're bored or just eating for pleasure.

If you plan to go out or be in environments where people around you are making poor choices, of course the odds are pretty high you're going to make bad choices. Stay out of the bad environment!

My weekends are almost always packed with fun outdoor activities. Plan an early morning hike with friends. Commit to a Saturday morning workout with someone. Plan activities that will make you want to go to bed early and get up early.

Here's what's going to happen. You're going to feel better all day long because you got up and did something active. You're going to save money because you didn't spend $100 on booze! You're going to feel great on Monday because you had such an active weekend! You're going to look better, feel better, and have more money. It's a no-brainer, if you ask me.

How Can I Get Rid of Belly Fat?

Unfortunately, you can't target fat loss. I know there are people selling products that claim, "Use this little ab machine to melt belly fat." It just doesn't work that way. I can show you how to make your bicep muscle bigger. But it's not possible to target fat loss from a specific body part. But that's okay, if you follow my plan, you'll lose fat everywhere.

Here is what I can tell you for sure. Improving strength and working the large muscle groups burns fat the fastest. That includes belly fat. Your leg and butt muscles are the big fat-burning furnaces in your body!

Is Coffee and Caffeine Good for Me?

Any pre-workout drink, any energy drink, all of them are just a way to get caffeine. The US consumes a ton of caffeine, and the overwhelming majority of it comes from Chinese chemical factories. The world's largest caffeine plant in China shipped 4.7 million pounds to the US in 2011.

The best energy drink is either an organic cup of coffee or tea. I highly recommend a device called the AeroPress. It makes amazing coffee and it takes a little bit of effort which helps to keep you from drinking too much. Coffee and tea both have health promoting properties that go along with the caffeine.

Don't get carried away with your coffee! If you're drinking a pot of coffee in the morning, a pot mid-morning, a pot for lunch, and just constantly sucking down coffee, that's not good. A couple cups per day are great.

As you become consistent with the plan I've given you in this book, you'll realize you need less coffee. You'll have more energy, wake up feeling fresher and need less caffeine throughout your day.

NO CAFFEINATED DRINKS FOR KIDS! The American Academy of Pediatrics stated that "rigorous review and analysis of the literature reveal that caffeine and other stimulant substances contained in energy drinks have no place in the diet of children and adolescents" (Schneider and Benjamin 2011). I cringe every time I see a kid with a bottle of sugar and caffeine, also known as soda.

Is Corn a Vegetable?

NO, it is NOT! How do you make a cow fat? Take away access to exercise and feed it corn. Corn is a grain and for fast success, you need to eliminate grains as much as possible.

How Big Is a Serving Size?

Portion control is extremely important! On average, American meal portions are enormous. A rather small meal, according to American standards, is still quite large. Even if you are eating less than the people around you, odds are you're still eating far too much. You have to be mindful of how much food you are eating. Here's the great news: when you eat less food, you save money!

When it comes to vegetables, you can eat as much as you want! I have yet to meet a person that is overweight because of a broccoli addiction. If you are still hungry after a meal, just eat more vegetables.

When it comes to healthy meats, a serving size would be the size of your palm. I wouldn't have more than one or two servings per meal. For fruits, as long as it's the whole fruit, I wouldn't worry too much about overeating. I have also yet to meet a person struggling with weight issues because of eating too many apples. That being said, I wouldn't recommend trying to pack down a whole watermelon. You'll have to pee 17 times that night and it has a lot of sugar.

Fruit	Fistful = 1 Cup	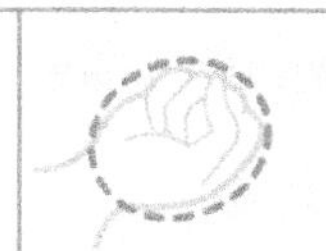
Fish and meats	Palm = 3.5 to 4 oz.	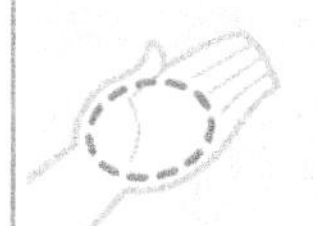
Trail mix, nuts, seeds	Handful = 1/4 cup	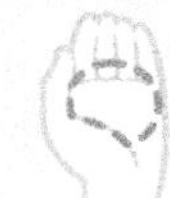
Veggies	2 Giant handfuls = Eat as much as you want!	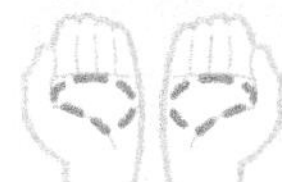
Oils, nut butters	Thumb = 1 oz.	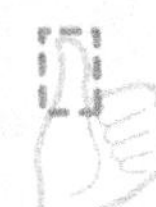

Where you really need to be careful is with nuts and oils. These high calorie, healthy foods can still put on fat. Think about animals that live in the wild and have no options other than healthy foods. They are still able to put on fat for the winter months. They actively search out the high-calorie nuts just so they can put on a layer of fat. You really have to be careful with portions here. For nuts and oils, a serving is about the size of your thumb. It's a much smaller amount than you might think but this is a must!

What If I'm Still Hungry?

When you eat less than your body is accustomed to, you may feel hungry. That feeling will pass. Hunger does not mean we need more food. Brush your teeth, drink a bunch of water, go do something active. Occupy your mind with other thoughts to block out the hunger. Your body will use your stored fat for energy. Some people have enough fat stores they could literally go an entire year without a bite of food!

Can I Eat Carbs?

Review the section in Chapter 5 on carbs. The secret is in choosing good carbs over bad carbs.

Should I Use Artificial Sweeteners?

When it comes to any artificial foods, history has proven that they've always been a bad idea. Consider artificial fats (trans fats), for example. They have been an epic failure and killed countless people. Synthetic vitamins (artificial vitamins) have been shown to increase cancers. Artificial sugars, or artificial sweeteners, have been around for a very short period of time. The evidence isn't clear, but I guarantee you the future will show they are a bad idea.

Newer studies have shown artificial sweeteners damage the good bacteria in our gut. They may also increase hunger and the amount you eat. When you consume artificial sweeteners, the sweet taste and lack of calories fools your body. Normally, when you eat something sweet, a lot of sugar calories come with it. This sweetness with no calories causes hunger and you will eat more. I would highly recommend avoiding all artificial sweeteners.

Should I Use Protein Powders?

No! There is a very good chance you are already getting more protein than you need in your diet. There is no reason to add more and turn your pee into a protein drink! Review the section on protein in Chapter 5 for more details.

What about Depriving My Kids of Treats?

One of the dumbest responses I hear is when a parent restricts their kid from eating junk food and an onlooker says, "You're going to give him/her an eating disorder." There isn't a shred of evidence, common sense or logic that shows depriving a kid of toxic junk food leads to future eating disorders. It's complete nonsense.

What leads to eating disorders is promoting thin and skinny as opposed to promoting strong and healthy. When the goal is to be skinny or lose weight, a person can make unhealthy choices to reach that goal because there is no focus on health. When a person eats and exercises to be healthy, fat-loss goals are reached and maintained.

Ask any group of kids, "Raise your hand if you want to be healthy." Try and find one that won't raise their hand. I'll never view junk food as a treat nor will I ever view exercise as a punishment.

In our home, treats are fruit: watermelon, plums, berries, apples, you name it. Those fruits bring my kids as much pleasure as any piece of candy could and they are good for them!

What about Pre-Workout Drinks?

Any pre-workout drink is just caffeine with a bunch of fluff added to it for marketing purposes. For the healthiest pre-workout drink possible, I would get a good organic cup of coffee or a good organic espresso shot. Don't like coffee? A caffeine pill washed down with water will give you the same energy boost as any pre-workout drink.

What about Post-Workout Drinks?

Again, there's not a shred of evidence that post-workout drinks improve the results of an athlete. You may hear that you need a shake within 30 minutes of your workout to boost your metabolism or boost muscle gain but there's no evidence to support any of that; it's just purely marketing. My post-workout drink or meal is whatever I choose to eat next. It's that simple. When you work out, give it plenty of effort and work out hard. And whenever you get the chance to eat next, choose healthy foods. Keep it that simple.

Why Don't You Like Calorie Counting?

Because calorie counting doesn't make any sense! For one thing, the calories listed on a package of food are often very, very wrong. Two, the calories you eat do not equal the calories you absorb. You absorb different amounts of calories from different foods. Three, different types of calories have different effects on your hormones which affect fat storage and fat burning.

A much wiser approach is to focus on nutrient density. I try to eat foods that have the highest amount of nutrients per calorie. I make it really, really simple. All you have to do is follow my grocery list and meal plan.

What Is the Thermic Effect of Food?

Understanding this action is very important. It goes along with calorie counting. For example, suppose you eat 1,000 calories of steak, a big steak; 300 of those calories are going to be burned up during the digestion process. Steak is harder to digest, and your body burns calories doing so. If you eat 1,000 calories of spaghetti, noodles are extremely easy to digest. Very quickly, your body absorbs all 1,000 calories of the spaghetti.

When you stick to whole foods that are harder to digest, you absorb less calories per meal. You will absorb more nutrients and less calories per meal, which means a healthier body with less fat.

Saying Goodbye

I'm serious. Just say it: "Goodbye." Say it out loud. Say, "Goodbye. Goodbye to the old me." It feels good to say goodbye to the old you. This is it. This is your last day to be where you are right now. From here on out, you'll have the growth mindset. You will get better and better. Not tomorrow, not this weekend, not whenever. No bullshit excuses. Today's the day. Today's the day to start making changes. You're committing to applying the Dr. Czys Method learned from this book.

You will embrace this challenge. You will persist in the face of setbacks. You will view the effort you put in as a path to mastery. You are going to ignore any negative feedback. You will show no envy and find inspiration and happiness from the success of others.

You will go to the grocery store and buy what's on the list. You're going to bring it home and start eating the way I show you. You're going to throw all the junk out of the house. Don't lie to yourself. If it's there, you will eat it. You can try and put it out of sight. But you know it's there. You will find it and eat it. Get it out of the house and start today because today is the day you say goodbye to the unhealthy, unmotivated you, and start saying hello to a much happier, healthier, vibrant future you!

Go to www.drczys.com/freetrial to access a ton of free material that I couldn't fit in this book! I've provided video demonstrations showing you exactly how to prepare everything. This program is literally one step away from me doing your grocery shopping and coming to cook for you. This is also a great place to send family and friends to if they are more visual or audio learners.

Chapter 11: The "One Step Away from Me Coming to Cook for You" Meal Plan

The "Lose 5-7 Pounds in One Week" Grocery Shopping List

Be sure to visit www.drczys.com/freetrial to watch a video in which I go through and explain this grocery shopping list and meal plan in detail.

Vegetables:

- ☐ 2 rutabagas
- ☐ 4 sweet potatoes
- ☐ 4-5 sweet onions
- ☐ Fresh broccoli
- ☐ 1 pepper (red or green)
- ☐ 1 zucchini
- ☐ 1 spaghetti squash
- ☐ 2 bags of baby carrots
- ☐ 1 container mushrooms
- ☐ 2 tomatoes
- ☐ 1 cauliflower
- ☐ 2 bags organic spinach
- ☐ Garlic – Always have lots of garlic on hand!
- ☐ Celery
- ☐ Lettuce for 5-6 salads (I prefer arugula/spinach/mixed greens)
- ☐ Veggies for your 5-6 salads (organic if possible: tomatoes, mushrooms, peppers, cucumbers, onions, carrots, broccoli, cauliflower, etc.)
- ☐ SALAD HACK – Go to the salad bar at the grocery store and make 5-6 salads. You'll be stocked up and ready to go for the week! I'm serious about this. I honestly think it's less expensive than buying all the ingredients.

Fruits: (Organic If Affordable)

☐ Bananas – At least 7
☐ Apples – Bag full
☐ Any fruit you like that's on sale
☐ 4 Avocados
☐ Nutritional yeast (fridge at Co-op)
☐ For smoothies, your choice of frozen strawberries, blueberries, mangoes, pineapple, papaya, oranges (4-5 cups of fruit TOTAL)

Meat:

☐ 2 packs of chicken thighs; 8 total thighs. Go with the Amish Farm brand, if available.
☐ 1 lb. ground grass-fed beef or venison
☐ 1 or 2 packages of chicken breasts
☐ 1 whole raw chicken
☐ Nitrate/nitrite-free bacon

Eggs:

☐ 2 dozen (organic, free range, hormone/antibiotic free if possible)

Nuts and Seeds:

☐ Pecans, almonds, brazil nuts, pistachios, and walnuts. Always on hand and always raw. (A peanut is NOT a nut!)

Miscellaneous:

☐ Unrefined coconut oil
☐ Olive oil (California Olive Ranch is great)
☐ Balsamic vinegar (no high fructose corn syrup)
☐ Apple cider vinegar
☐ Bragg Liquid Aminos
☐ Bragg salad dressing if you don't want to make your own, any flavor
☐ Organic spaghetti sauce
☐ Dijon mustard (no corn syrup)
☐ For chocolate smoothies: Enrich from Eupraxia (optional)

Spices:

- ☐ Pink Himalayan sea or Celtic salt
- ☐ Freshly ground pepper
- ☐ Dried onion powder
- ☐ Garlic powder
- ☐ Thyme
- ☐ Basil
- ☐ Dried parsley
- ☐ Curry
- ☐ Dill weed
- ☐ Tarragon
- ☐ Cumin
- ☐ Cayenne or red pepper flakes
- ☐ Oregano
- ☐ Cinnamon

Fresh Herbs:

- ☐ Fresh dill weed

Tea and Coffee

- ☐ Green tea or other teas, organic if possible (optional)
- ☐ Coffee (for creamer: ONLY use coconut milk or almond milk or Enrich), NO sweetener (optional)

Supplements: These Are Incredibly Important – I NEVER Miss The Big Three

- ☐ Physics Nutrition Fish Oil: Take 1 gel cap per 50 lb. of body weight
- ☐ Physics Nutrition Vitamin D3
- ☐ Physics Nutrition Probiotics:
- ☐ Enrich: great for coffee and amazing smoothies (optional)

THE "IT'S SO SIMPLE, IF YOU'RE AT LEAST 12 AND CAN READ, YOU CAN DO IT" MEAL PLAN

All recipes for meals in this plan can be found in Chapter 12.

	Monday
Breakfast	Fried Eggs, 1 Apple
Snack	Choose a snack from my top 10 list
Lunch	Large Green Salad w/ veggies and 1 Tbs. Apple Cider Vinaigrette
Dinner	Baked Chicken Thighs with Broccoli Stir Fry (Marinate tomorrow's Chicken Breast)
Supplements	[Fish Oil + Vit D +Probiotics]

	Tuesday
Breakfast	Fried eggs, Leftover Broccoli Stir Fry
Snack	Choose a snack from my top 10 list
Lunch	Large Green Salad w/ veggies and 1 Tbs. Dressing of choice
Dinner	Marinated Chicken Breast with Cumin Cauliflower
Supplements	[Fish Oil + Vit D +Probiotics]

	Wednesday
Breakfast	Fried Eggs, 1 Apple
Snack	Choose a snack from my top 10 list
Lunch	Leftover Chicken Breast and Cauliflower
Dinner	Spaghetti Squash and Meat Sauce
Supplements	[Fish Oil + Vit D +Probiotics]

	Thursday
Breakfast	Strawberry Banana Smoothie
Snack	Choose a snack from my top 10 list
Lunch	Large Green Salad w/ veggies and 1 Tbs. Dressing of choice
Dinner	Veggie Stir Fry with Leftover Chicken
Supplements	[Fish Oil + Vit D +Probiotics]

	Friday
Breakfast	Fried Eggs with Leftover Veggie Stir Fry
Snack	Choose a snack from my top 10 list
Lunch	Leftover Spaghetti Squash and Meat Sauce
Dinner	Baked Whole Chicken and Mixed Veggies
Supplements	[Fish Oil + Vit D +Probiotics]

	Saturday
Breakfast	Egg Muffins
Snack	Choose a snack from my top 10 list
Lunch	Leftover Baked Chicken and Mixed Vegetables
Dinner	Mom's Chicken Soup
Supplements	[Fish Oil + Vit D +Probiotics]

	Sunday
Breakfast	Lazy Egg Scramble
Snack	Choose a snack from my top 10 list
Lunch	Leftover Mom's Chicken Soup
Dinner	Go to www.drczys.com/freetrial and get meal plans for12 more weeks!
Supplements	[Fish Oil + Vit D +Probiotics]

CAN I EAT_____? ANSWERS TO ALL OF YOUR FOOD QUESTIONS

If it's not in this list, it's not something I would recommend! If you just follow these rules and only buy the foods listed, you will look and feel better. The specifics behind why a food may not be listed can be found on the membership site. The more time you spend on that site, the better your results will be!

When it comes to the health of me and my family, the goal is OPTIMAL! If something is only "pretty good," that won't cut it. If you don't see something on this list, you won't find it in my home.

The goal is to make all of this as easy as possible for you! I have NEVER heard from anyone who followed this advice that he/she didn't feel better.

The Three Basic Changes

There is a ton of misinformation out there when it comes to nutrition advice. Why? Money. Influencers are hired and a lot of nutrition advice is focused more on selling a product than what is actually healthy for you. Recently, it was revealed that 50 years ago, Harvard doctors were flat out paid to write articles vilifying all fats and claiming sugar was good. Those docs were literally paid to lie.

The first two changes are very simple to implement because they are horizontal shifts in your eating habits. If you are eating manmade fats and unhealthy meats, simply replace them with healthy fats and meats. This takes very little effort, other than becoming educated about your new food choices listed below.

The third change is a bit more challenging but will yield the greatest results. Unwanted body fat will melt away! This change may be difficult, but it will lead to the greatest transformation in your health and well-being.

I have observed the best results when people just went all in! Tell yourself today you are going all in. Six weeks from now, the average person will have lost 20-25 pounds. You'll be amazed at how much your body has changed. In a year, you can be a completely different person!

1. Remove the BAD FATS and Replace them with HEALTHY FATS.

- Bad fats such as hydrogenated and partially hydrogenated oils, trans fats, and rancid vegetable oils are poisons that make you fat and have killed hundreds of thousands of people. You won't see any listed below.
- Healthy fats are the nutrients most lacking in the standard American diet (SAD), not vitamins and minerals (i.e., fish oil!).
- Healthy fats are essential to hormone production, cancer prevention, brain development, weight loss, cellular healing, and reducing inflammation.
- Coconut oil, olive oil, and avocado oil – The only three oils you should have in your home! Just throw the rest away.
- Vegetable oil – Look at the ingredients; they're never vegetables but always a grain or legume. Clever marketing! Throw it out!

2. Change the MEATS that you EAT.

- It doesn't really matter what type of animal the meat comes from. What matters is how that animal was raised.
- Animals meant to eat grass are often fed grains to fatten them up faster. These animals produce more unhealthy fat and less healthy fat. You end up lacking healthy fat and eating loads of pro-inflammatory unhealthy fat, making you fatter and sicker.
- The bioaccumulation of commercial pesticides, herbicides, antibiotics, and hormones in meats is devastating to health. This leads to many cancers and chronic illness.
- Grass-fed, wild, and free-range meats offer many fats missing in the standard American diet, such as omega-3 fatty acids.
- Use meat from un-medicated wild or grass-fed animals only!
- The most cost-effective strategy is to buy quality meat in bulk from an organic farmer. Fill up a chest freezer once and eat for months! SAVE TIME AND MONEY!

3. Remove ALL refined SUGARS, GRAINS, and DAIRY from your diet (The Harder Part).

- This includes rice, pasta and bread. I know it may sound impossible, but you'll be amazed how good you feel once you do this!
- One third of sugar intake comes from soft drinks, two thirds from hidden sources, including: lunch meats, pizza, sauces, breads, soups, crackers, fruit drinks, canned foods, yogurt, etc.
- Added sugar is an anti-nutrient, offering insignificant amounts of vitamins and minerals and robbing your body of precious nutrient stores. This inevitably leads to today's common diseases, such as obesity, faster aging, chronic fatigue, ADD, ADHD, heart disease, diabetes, and cancers.
- Sugar is devastating to your immune system.
- Corn is not a vegetable and should be avoided as much as possible. This includes all high fructose corn syrup. How do you make cows gain weight? Feed them corn!
- Grains like wheat and corn should be avoided as much as possible.
- Cow milk is for baby cows, not humans! Use almond or coconut milk. I discuss this in Chapter 6 and on my membership site.

Food Choices

If it's not listed below, I wouldn't buy it!

HEALTHY PROTEIN CHOICES

Choose grass-fed, free-range, cage-free, and no-hormones-added sources whenever possible. Avoid farm-raised fish.

- Cold water fish - salmon, sardines, mahi-mahi, mackerel, etc.
- Eggs (local, farmer-raised, if possible)
- Chicken and turkey
- Venison
- Wild game meats
- Beef
- Lamb
- Game birds: pheasant, duck, goose, grouse, turkey, etc.

HEALTHY FAT CHOICES

Choose raw instead of roasted nuts, if possible. Oils should be cold pressed and unrefined.

- Raw nuts and seeds: almonds, cashews, flax, hemp, pecans, pine nuts, macadamia, sesame, sunflower, walnuts, etc.
- Grass-fed meat
- Coconut or flakes
- Fish oil
- Hemp oil (3 to 1 ratio)
- Olive oil, olives
- Flaxseed oil
- Grape seed oil
- Almond butter
- Avocado
- Organic raw animal butter
- Avocado oil
- Coconut milk, oil, and butter
- Eggs (local, farmer-raised, if possible)

Note: AVOID hydrogenated and partially hydrogenated oils, such as cottonseed oil, soybean oil, canola oil, and vegetable oils; trans fats such as margarine and synthetic butters; rancid vegetable oils such as corn oil, canola oil, or those labeled simply vegetable oil, found in practically every bread, cracker, cookie, and boxed food product.

VEGETABLE CHOICES

Choose organic when possible but know that a conventional vegetable is far better than the conventional grains! You don't have to buy all organic if cost is an issue. Remember, all fruits and vegetables are carbs!

Artichokes	Broad beans	Chayote fruit
Arugula	Broccoli	Chicory
Asparagus	Carrots	Chives
Bamboo shoots	Cassava	Collard greens

Bean sprouts	Cauliflower	Coriander
Beet greens	Celery	Dandelion greens
Brussel sprouts	Kohlrabi	Radicchio
Cabbage	Leeks	Shallots
Eggplant	Lettuce	Snap beans
Endive	Mushrooms	Spinach
Fennel	Kohlrabi	Sweet potato
Garlic	Mustard greens	Swiss chard
Ginger root	Onions	Turnip greens
Hearts of Palm	Parsley	Turnip
Jicama (raw)	Pumpkin	Watercress
Kale	Radishes	

Fruit choices

- Choose organic when possible. If weight loss is a concern, try to go heavier on the veggies than fruits.
- Organic is most important for fruits that you don't peel but actually eat the skin.
- Fruit juice is NOT a good choice. It's just sugar water.

Best fruit choices, especially if weight loss is a concern: Berries

(blackberries, blueberries, boysenberries, elderberries, gooseberries, loganberries, raspberries, strawberries)

Fresh fruit is always your dessert and treat of choice! More approved fruits:

Cherries	Tangerines	Plums
Pears	Passion fruits	Grapefruit
Fresh apricots	Persimmons	Pitted prunes
Pomegranates	Papaya	Apples

Melons	Bananas	Avocados
Oranges	Pineapple	Kiwi fruits
Peaches	Grapes	Lemons
Limes	Bell peppers	Squash
Nectarines	Tomatoes	Spaghetti squash
Watermelon	Jalapeno peppers	Summer squash
Mangos	Cucumbers	

Cooking and Eating Tips

- Removing grains and refined sugars is easiest when removed completely and all at once. Your body will adapt to the change quickly and cravings will diminish in approximately 1 ½ weeks.
- Be sure to drink only clean water (not city tap water) when thirsty. Reverse osmosis (RO) and/or distilled water are best. The only thing you need to drink is water and your body tells you when you need it via thirst. It really is that simple.
- Heathy fats like eggs, avocadoes, or nuts for breakfast helps people eat less the rest of the day.
- Have healthy snacks available for snacking at all times. It's wise to have healthy options available.
- Moderation is key, do not eat until you are stuffed. If you are looking to lose weight, you must have the discipline to watch portion sizes.
- PURGE! If you shouldn't eat it, get it out of your house. It is much easier to make bad choices if the food is just sitting in the cupboard. If you have to make a trip to the store to satisfy a craving, you are much less likely to do it. Willpower is like a muscle; you can wear it out.
- Plan ahead! People most often "cheat" when they are in a hurry and need something fast. Plan ahead and have healthy food available.

Tip 1: How to cook with fats and oils

- High heat: The best choice for high heat is avocado oil because of its high smoke point.
- Medium heat: To sauté foods, use coconut oil or avocado oil. Animal fats work great as well. I'll often use rendered deer fat or the grease I save from cooked bacon.
- Baking: Organic butter, coconut oil, or olive oil can be used in baking if the temperature is less than 325° F. In a hotter oven, I would use avocado oil or animal fats.
- Low or no heat: Extra virgin cold-pressed olive oil is amazing.

Tip 2: Eat more vegetables

A sweet potato is a better option than a white potato because of high nutrient content and they are sprayed far less. Be sure to always get organic potatoes. If you want to lose fat fast, try to limit consumption of any potato.

- Corn is not a vegetable; it is a grain and should be avoided.
- A peanut is not a nut, it is a legume. Avoid cheap peanut butter. Almond butter is a great option.
- Listen to your body. Your cravings and energy levels will tell you when you need to adjust or modify your personal plan. However, during the first two weeks, while insulin levels are adjusting, you will feel extra hungry. You need to have willpower!

Tip 3: Eliminating added sugar is critical

- Refined sugar lowers the immune system.
- Sugar promotes the growth of bad bacteria in your mouth and gut. Cavities are no fun.
- One can of soda has 9 to 11 teaspoons of sugar.
- Today, Americans consume 57 pounds of sugar per year in contrast to the early 1900s when they consumed only 5 per family in a year.
- Avoid corn syrup, fructose, large amounts of honey or molasses, sucrose, maltodextrin, dextrose, any artificial sweeteners, fruit juices and syrups, sugar cane, and lactose
- The stevia herb is an acceptable sweetener.

Recommended Supplements

The first three supplements listed are an absolute must. My family takes them, and they are all available for purchase at https://drczys.com/myproducts/. If you are not getting enough of these nutrients in your diet, you cannot be fully healthy. There is a huge difference in quality between supplements. I cover this in detail in Chapter 7 and on the membership site. Be sure to review that section! These first three supplements are most important for kids, as well.

Physics Nutrition Fish Oil

1 capsule per day per 50 lb. of body weight.

A liquid version is available for adults and kids as well.

Physics Nutrition Probiotic

1 capsule per day for those without digestive issues.

2 capsules per day until digestive issues subside.

This product is suitable for kids. Just open the capsule and add the powder to their food.

Physics Nutrition Vitamin D3

Available in capsules for adults and liquid drops for kids.

Enrich

A great way to get extra fruits, veggies, and fiber in your diet. It makes amazing, healthy smoothies.

Physics Nutrition Mother Nature's Multi Vitamin

1 per day per 50 lb. of body weight.

Bonus: U-Tract (D-Mannose)

Great for urinary tract infections. This product has worked for every patient I've seen with a UTI. The UTI will be gone within two days. Very rarely would you need to take an antibiotic.

YOU ARE AN ACTION TAKER!

Here's the truth. I've never met a person who has applied what you've just read and regretted it. Every single one is happier after making the lifestyle changes and has started looking and feeling better.

Unfortunately, I have also talked to many who are full of regret for not making the changes earlier and wish they had taken action.

You are the person who will take action! I highly recommend taking your "before" pictures today!! You will not believe the visible changes after a few weeks when you compare them to your "after" pictures!

Lastly, I want you to know that I truly appreciate you; taking the time to read this book means a lot to me. If you have found value in and enjoyed the information and advice I've shared, the greatest compliment you could give is to recommend it to others. It's time to let everyone in on the secret of the "cheat code" truth!

Steps to Take Today

LEVEL ONE

Join my online program at www.drczys.com/freebies. I did my best to create a program that makes switching to an enjoyable, healthy lifestyle as simple as possible for you. The best thing you can do is just go to the site and see everything that's in it. It's exactly what you've been hoping for!

LEVEL TWO

Join Eupraxia! This takes it to the next level; it's the online program on steroids. At Eupraxia, you'll be able to do all the workouts I created with an amazing group of people. Expert trainers will be there every single day making sure you do everything properly.

You'll get the entire "one step from me coming and cooking for you" nutrition program that every other fitness program is missing. You'll have an "accountabilibuddy" to hold you accountable and ensure you apply the program. And you'll have loads of fun in the process. Join at www.eupraxia.us.

Level three

If you absolutely love helping others and want to reach for the highest level, you can apply to open a Eupraxia of your own. I will teach you everything necessary to transform lives in your community. In my opinion, there is nothing more satisfying than making a living through improving the lives of others. I wake up every single day excited to go to "work." You can apply at www.eupraxia.us.

Chapter 12: Recipes for Celebration!

Fried Eggs and Fruit

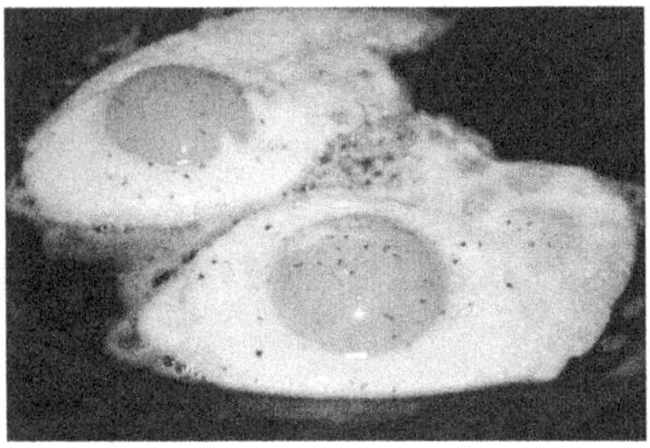

I start just about every day with eggs. I'm going to change the mornings up for you. However, if you love eggs and how easy it is to make them, you can have them every day.

Ingredients:

- 2-6 eggs – cooked how you like.
- Olive oil
- Salt and pepper
- (Optional) Don't be afraid to try different seasonings on eggs. Curry is great. Tarragon is great.
- 1 apple

Directions: Heat frying pan to low/medium heat.

Add a little bit of olive oil, your eggs, and your seasonings. As they are cooking, cut up your apple. In about five minutes, you have a wonderful, healthy breakfast.

Apple Cider Vinegar Dressing

I keep a bottle of this in the fridge at all times!

Ingredients:

- 1 cup extra virgin olive oil
- 1/2 cup apple cider vinegar
- 1 tsp. dried onion powder
- 2 Tbsp. Dijon mustard
- 2 garlic cloves, passed through a garlic press or minced (optional)
- 1/2 tsp. sea salt
- 1/2 tsp. of dried thyme
- 1/2 tsp. of dried basil
- Freshly ground pepper, to taste

Directions: Add all ingredients into a bowl and whisk until thoroughly combined.

Salad
Fresh and Healthy!

Make it HUGE.

Ingredients:

- Whatever veggies you'd like. You seriously can't eat too many fresh veggies. Load it up and enjoy. I like mixed greens, baby spinach, mushrooms, olives, hot peppers, pickled beets, cilantro, broccoli, cauliflower, tomatoes, peppers, and cucumber; pretty much anything.
- Often, I prefer to just make a few salads at the grocery store salad bar. You do what works best for you!

Directions: Mix it up, top with your dressing of choice and enjoy.

Baked Chicken Thighs

I make baked chicken thighs every week.

Ingredients:

- Chicken thighs
- Salt and pepper
- Curry
- Any seasoning you'd like! Download a load of free spice mixes at www.drczys.com/freetrial

Directions: Preheat the oven to 350°F.

Put the thighs (thawed) on a baking dish, skin side up. Season with salt and pepper and go heavy on the curry or any other seasoning you'd like.

Bake at 350° for about 55 minutes. The crispy skin is almost too good! A small purchase I recommend and absolutely love is a digital meat thermometer. The thermometer will beep at exactly 165 degrees so your chicken will always be cooked to perfection!

Favorite Broccoli Stir Fry

This is one of my fav go-to recipes for a side dish. It's so EASY and delish!

Ingredients:

- Broccoli (enough to fill a BIG frying pan or stir fry pan). Cut into florets. If you want to use the stems, cut into bite-sized pieces. I use the whole stem, too.
- Extra virgin olive oil
- Bragg Liquid Aminos
- Pepper if you'd like. Pepper makes everything better

Directions: Make this while your chicken is baking.

Pour a little olive oil into your pan. Cut up enough broccoli to fill that pan. Add about 2 Tablespoons of Bragg Liquid Aminos and stir fry on the stovetop until the broccoli is soft. Set the heat on medium, put the cover on the pan, and stir up the veggies every few minutes. Just keep the broccoli from burning and sticking to the bottom. When you can easily stab the broccoli with a fork, it is done. If you want more flavor, just add a little more Bragg Liquid Aminos to it.

You made a lot of veggies. The extras are for breakfast!

Note: You can add any veggies you like to this! Carrots, mushrooms, cauliflower, parsnips, Brussels sprouts, asparagus, water chestnuts, etc. Change it up and discover what you love!

Easy Breezy Marinated Chicken Breast

Makes 6-8 servings

Feel free to make a LOT. Chicken is always good to have on hand for salads and lettuce wraps.

Ingredients:

- Chicken breasts
- 1/2 cup lemon juice
- 3 cloves garlic, minced
- 2 tsp. olive oil
- 2 tsp. tarragon
- 1 tsp. thyme
- 3/4 tsp. salt
- 2 tsp. black pepper

Directions: In a one-gallon plastic Ziploc bag, combine lemon juice, garlic, olive oil, tarragon, thyme, salt and pepper.

Add chicken breasts to the bag and make sure they are all coated evenly with marinade. Squeeze the air out of the bag and seal it.

Marinate the chicken in the refrigerator for at least 1-2 hours, turning over occasionally.

Preheat the oven to 350°F. Place the chicken breasts in a glass baking dish. Bake covered in aluminum foil for about 10 minutes, and then UNCOVER and cook for about 10 minutes more or until juices run clear. This would be a great time to use the digital meat thermometer!

Cumin Cauliflower

Ingredients:

- 1 entire head of cauliflower, chopped into small pieces. (remove leaves)
- Olive oil
- Cumin
- Sea salt and pepper to taste

Directions: In a medium pot, add the olive oil, spices and cauliflower. Cover and cook on medium. If you need to add more olive oil while it's cooking, go ahead. Make sure your pot doesn't run dry. Mix it up occasionally to keep it from burning. When it's fork tender, it is ready. Save some for lunch tomorrow!

Enjoy.

Spaghetti Squash and Meat Sauce

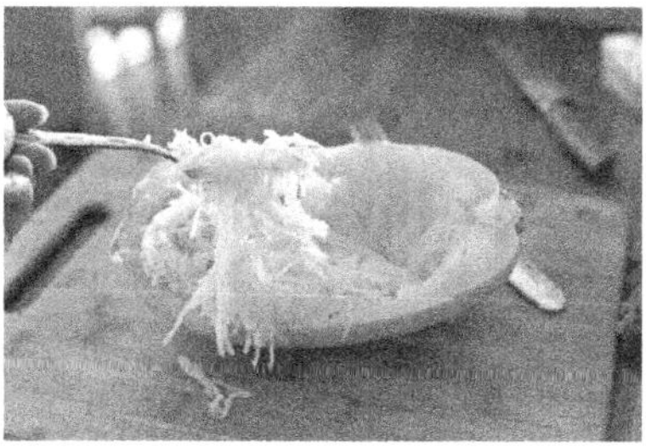

Ingredients:

- 1 Spaghetti squash, cut in half length-wise, and de-seeded
- Extra virgin olive oil
- Ground grass-fed beef or venison
- Sea salt and fresh ground pepper to taste

Directions: Preheat your oven to 400°F. Cover a baking pan in aluminum foil and set aside.

Place the two halves of de-seeded squash, insides facing UP, in the pan, and put the pan in the oven. Cook for 45-60 minutes. If you squeeze the squash and it's still hard, cook it longer.

Once it cools a bit, use a fork to "shred" and pull out the spaghetti squash. It comes out like spaghetti—pretty awesome!

While the squash is cooking, add a little olive oil and ground meat to a frying pan. Cook on low/medium heat until browned. Add a jar of spaghetti sauce to the meat once it has been browned. Top the spaghetti squash with sauce and enjoy!

Bonus Recipe: If you have extra spaghetti squash, place a small pile of it in a frying pan with a little olive oil, salt and pepper and have spaghetti squash hash browns with your eggs!

Strawberry-Banana Morning Blast

Ingredients:

- 1 cup water
- 1 cup strawberries (or frozen mixed berries)
- 1/3 banana
- 1-2 cups spinach

Quick Tip: Blend the water with the greens FIRST, and then add the rest of the ingredients. Makes 1 serving.

How to Hard Boil an Egg

Ingredients:

4-6 eggs (you can make as many as you want at the same time)

Directions:

Place eggs in a large pot. Fill the pot with cool water to one inch above the eggs. Bring water to a boil over high heat. When the water reaches a boil, set the timer for the desired time. Boil for 6-7 minutes over medium to high heat. Keep track of the time and how your eggs turn out. Eventually you'll figure out a perfect length of time.

Immediately put the eggs in ice water! This is the secret to easy peeling. You can even crack them a bit in the water, so a little water will get under the shell. This makes peeling even easier.

Veggie Stir Fry

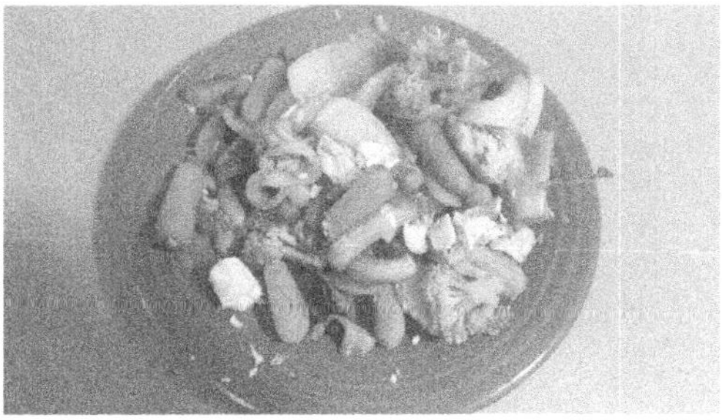

Ingredients:

- Any vegetable of choice, cut to bite-sized pieces (broccoli, cauliflower, asparagus, carrots, onions or other vegetable of choice)
- 1 TBSP olive oil
- 2 TBSP Bragg Liquid Aminos

Directions: Add your veggies, olive oil and liquid aminos to a large frying or stir fry pan. Cover and cook on medium heat, occasionally stirring. When they are fork tender, they are done. Eat as much as you want! Learn to LOVE your veggies.

I like to add my veggies stir fry to a plate full of mixed greens. Make sure there is extra for the morning!

Fried Eggs and Veggies

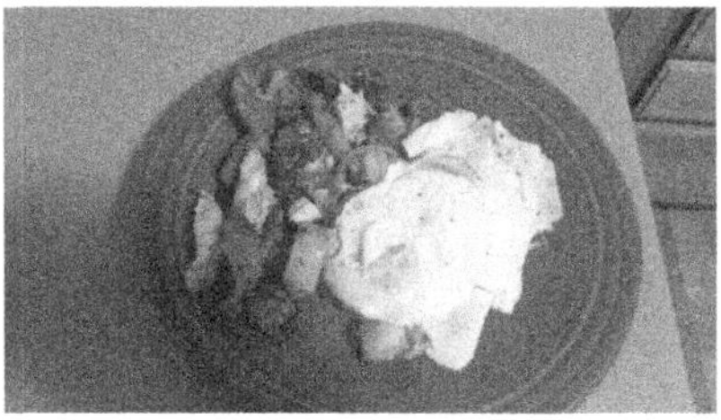

Ingredients:

- Eggs
- Broccoli, carrots, mixed veggies, etc.

Directions: So good and so easy! Last night's leftovers with today's eggs!

Baked Whole Chicken and Mixed Veggies

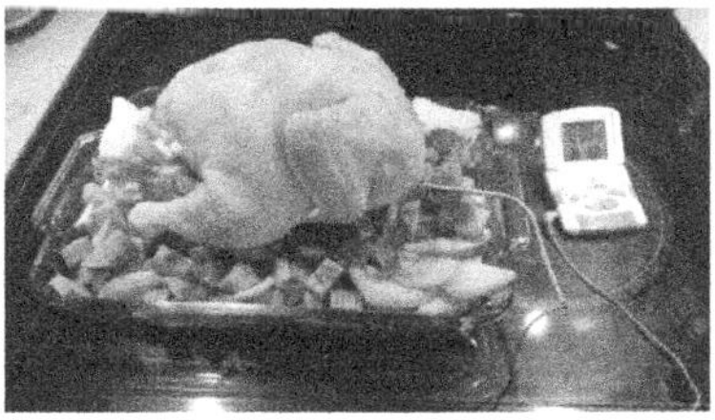

Ingredients:

- 1 whole chicken
- 2 parsnips, cut into bite-sized pieces
- 1 onion, diced
- 1 apple, cut into chunks
- 1 sweet potato, cubed
- 1 rutabaga, peeled and cubed
- 1/2 cup carrots peeled and cut in pieces
- 2-3 Tablespoons dill weed
- Sea salt and black pepper to taste

Directions: In a large baking dish, add any combo of the veggies listed above. You can use whatever you'd like. Just fill up the dish.

Cover with a healthy dose of dill weed, salt and pepper. Put the chicken on top and bake at 350°F for about 75 minutes. A digital thermometer (see photo) beeps when the meat is at the perfect temperature. You never have to worry about dried out or undercooked chicken.

The juices from the chicken leak out and add great flavor to your veggies.

Save the chicken bones to make bone broth to use with the Mom's Chicken Soup recipe. A video showing how easy it is to make bone broth can be viewed at www.drczys.com/freetrial.

Egg Muffins

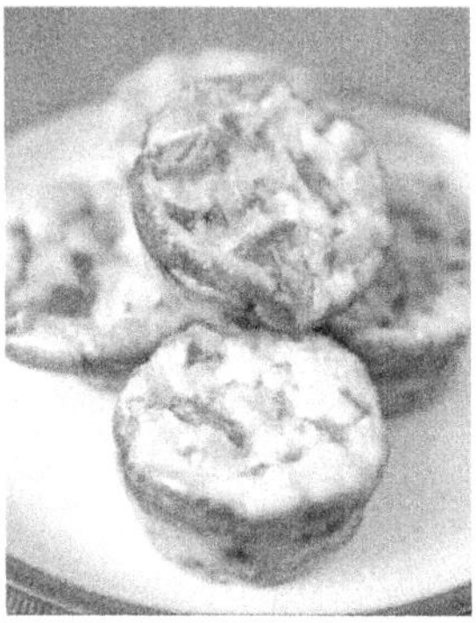

Cook once and store in the refrigerator for easy breakfast all week. These also make a great back-up breakfast during the week if you're in a rush as well as a great snack alternative.

Ingredients:

- 12 eggs
- 1/2 onion, diced
- 1 fresh red pepper, seeded and diced
- 1 zucchini, diced
- 6 slices of bacon/turkey bacon (nitrate-free)
- 4 cups fresh spinach
- Fresh ground pepper to taste

Directions: Preheat oven to 350°F, and lightly grease 2 muffin tins with coconut oil.

In a medium sauté pan, heat coconut oil and sauté onions for 3-4 minutes until softened. Add pepper and sauté for another 2-3 minutes until the pepper has softened. Drain any excess oil and set aside.

In a food processor, process the zucchini and bacon until finely chopped.

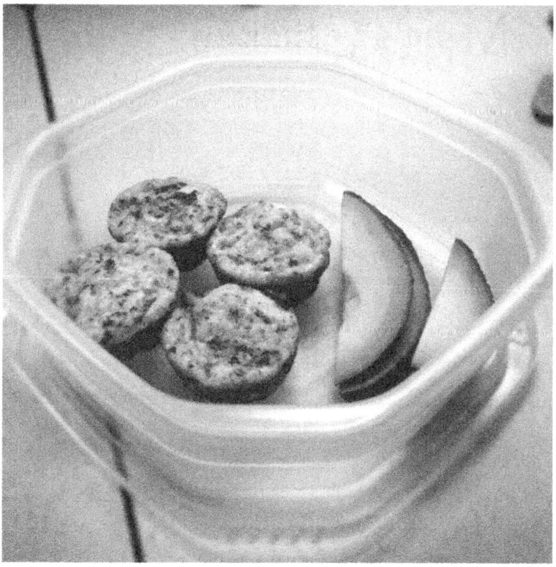

Whisk the 12 eggs and season with pepper. Mix your zucchini and bacon mixture in with your eggs.

Then, finely chop the 4 cups of spinach in the processor and add these to your eggs in the bowl. Add the onion and pepper mixture to your eggs.

Mix the egg mixture thoroughly and fill muffin tins with ¼ cup of your mixture. Bake for 20-25 minutes or until the egg-muffins have set in the middle.

Mom's Chicken Soup

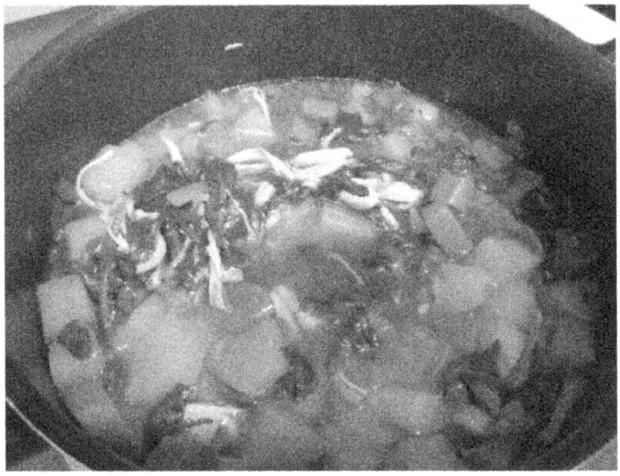

Ingredients:

- 2 chicken breasts on the bone, skin removed
- 1 onion, quartered and then sliced into ¼-inch slices
- 2 celery stalks, rinsed and sliced into ¼-inch pieces
- 3 carrots, peeled, and sliced into ½-inch pieces
- 1 rutabaga, peeled and cubed
- 1 bunch fresh dill, rinsed
- Sea salt and pepper to taste
- 2-3 Tbsp. olive oil
- 1 pound of baby spinach

Directions:

Heat olive oil in a large heavy stockpot. Set on medium heat, put in the chicken and lightly brown on top and bottom. Remove from pot and add onions.

Season onions with salt and pepper and cook until tender and lightly golden. Return chicken to the pot and add enough chicken broth or water to cover chicken, and then about one inch higher.

Bring to a boil and add all the vegetables, including the dill. Bring to a simmer and cook with the pot half covered for about 30 minutes, or until all the vegetables are fork tender. Turn off the heat.

Remove the chicken and let cool until you are able to handle it with your hands. Remove the dill.

Shred the chicken and return it to the pot. Season the broth with salt and pepper. Add the spinach. The heat from the soup will cook the spinach. If you like, you can put some sliced avocado on top. AMAZING!

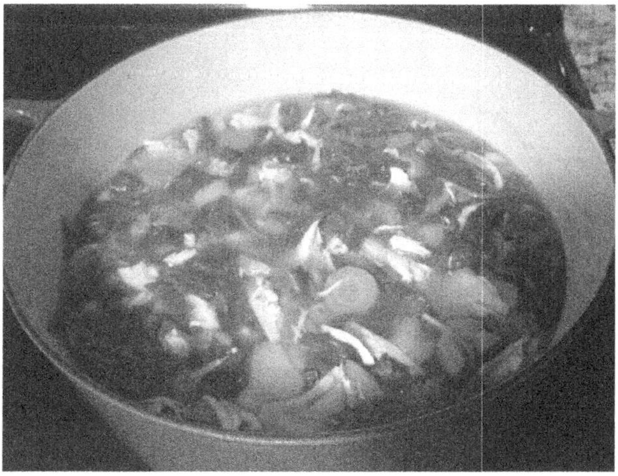

Lazy Egg Scramble

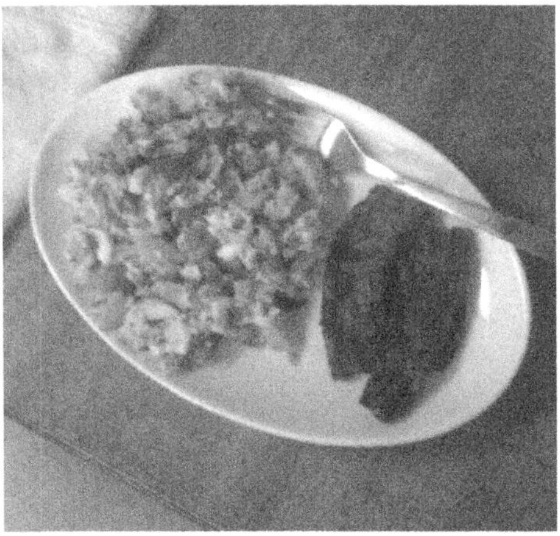

If you prep the veggies ahead of time, this is an excellent and FAST breakfast during the week. **Make a whole bunch of extra veggies!**

Prep ahead of time to save time later. Makes 4-6 servings once you add the eggs.

Ingredients:

- 1-2 Tbsp. olive oil
- 1 lb. spinach
- Sea salt and freshly ground pepper
- Any veggies you have in the house! (about 2-4 cups total depending on how much you want to make) I use chopped sweet onion, red pepper, tomato, mushrooms, but you can use any veggies you want; green pepper, artichoke, etc.

Directions: Place a large sauté pan on medium heat. Place a bunch of spinach into the pan. With tongs, gently continue tossing until the spinach has wilted (1 minute).

Don't leave the spinach in the pan, it will burn! As soon as it's finished wilting, remove spinach and place on a plate and repeat with the rest of the spinach.

Next, heat up a little olive oil and sauté onions for a few minutes BEFORE adding the other chopped veggies to the pan. Season with salt and pepper. Sauté all the veggies to your liking (about a few minutes).

Add spinach to the sauté mixture. Let cool for a few minutes and then store in a storage container for up to a week in the fridge.

(I usually make a BIG batch of this once a week and add this to my eggs throughout the week when I don't make a green smoothie.)

To complete the Scramble:

- 1/2 tsp. olive oil
- 2-3 eggs, whisked in a bowl
- Sea salt and fresh ground pepper for seasoning

In a medium sauté pan, heat olive oil over low/med heat. Add the eggs and season with salt and pepper. Stir and then let sit until nearly set. Add your desired amount of sautéed veggies to the eggs. (I like a LOT of veggies and will put about a 1/2 to 1 cup of veggies in mine.

Continue to mix eggs until cooked. Serve hot and enjoy!

Popcorn Snack

Ingredients:

- 1 TBSP coconut oil
- 1/2 cup popcorn seeds, plus a few more
- Olive oil
- Salt
- Nutritional yeast
- Other seasonings, if you'd like

Add a Tablespoon of coconut oil and a **few** popcorn seeds to a large pot. Place it on the stove top and turn the burner to medium.

Once those seeds pop, add 1/2 cup of popcorn seeds and put the cover on a little loosely to allow steam to escape.

Give the pan a shake a few times while the seeds are popping.

Once the pops are few and far between, remove from heat and pour popcorn into a bowl.

Now for the fun part! My favorite way to season is with olive oil, salt and nutritional yeast. The nutritional yeast adds a great nutty cheese flavor.

You can also add balsamic vinegar, hot sauce, taco seasoning...play around and have fun!

Watch my video "Popcorn Perfected" to see how I demonstrate this recipe (YouTube channel: Dr Steve Czys).

References

Afshin, A., P. Sur, K. Fay, G. Ferra, E. Mullany, C. Murray, S. Biryukov, et al. 2019. "Health effects of dietary risks in 195 countries, 1990–2017: a systematic analysis for the Global Burden of Disease Study 2017." *The Lancet.*

Ahmad, A. S., N. Ormiston-Smith, and P. D. Sasieni. 2015. "Trends in the lifetime risk of developing cancer in Great Britain: comparison of risk for those born from 1930 to 1960." *British Journal of Cancer* 943–947.

Åkerblom, Hans K., Mikael Knip, and Suvi M. Virtanen. 2010. "Infant feeding and the risk of type 1 diabetes." *The American Journal of Clinical Nutrition* 1506S–1513S.

Atlas, Family Health Center. 2017. *Still Drinking Milk? (May 2010).* August 15. Accessed March 2019. https://atlasfamilyhealthcenter.com/still-drinking-milk-may-2010/.

Bertron, P., N. D. Barnard, and M. Mills. 1999. "Racial bias in federal nutrition policy, Part I: The public health implications of variations in lactase persistence." *Journal of the National Medical Association* 151–157.

Bertron, RD, Patricia, MD, Neal D. Barnard, and MD, Milton Mills. 1999. "Racial bias in federal nutrition policy, part 1: The public health implications of variations in lactase persistence." *Journal of the National Medical Association* 151-157.

Bischoff-Ferrari, Heike A., Bess Dawson-Hughes, John A. Baron, Peter Burckhardt, Ruifeng Li, Donna Spiegelman, Bonny Specker, et al. 2007. "Calcium intake and hip fracture risk in men and women: a meta-analysis of prospective cohort studies and randomized controlled trials." *The American Journal of Clinical Nutrition* 1780–1790.

Cho, Karl, Tommy Cederholm, and Johan Lökk. 2008. "Calcium intake in elderly patients with hip fractures." *Food & Nutrition Research.*

Copley, M. S., R. Berstan, S. N. Dudd, G. Docherty, A. J. Mukherjee, V. Straker, S. Payne, and R. P. Evershed. 2003. "Direct chemical evidence for widespread dairying in prehistoric Britain." *Proceedings of the National Academy of Sciences of the USA* 1524-1529.

Cordain, Loren, L. Toohey, M. J. Smith, and M. S. Hickey. 2007. "Modulation of immune function by dietary lectins in rheumatoid arthritis." *British Journal of Nutrition* 207-217.

Farlow, Daniel W., Xia Xu, and Timothy D. Veenstra. 2009. "Quantitative measurement of endogenous estrogen metabolites, risk-factors for development of breast cancer, in commercial milk products by LC–MS/MS." *Journal of Chromatography B* 1327-1334.

Hill, Alison M., Jonathan D. Buckley, Karen J. Murphy, and Peter RC Howe. 2007. "Combining fish-oil supplements with regular aerobic exercise improves body composition and cardiovascular disease risk factors." *the American Journal of Clinical Nutrition* 1267–1274.

Holmes, Michelle D., Michael N. Pollak, Walter C. Willett, and Susan E. Hankinson. 2002. "Dietary Correlates of Plasma Insulin-like Growth Factor I and Insulin-like Growth Factor Binding Protein 3 Concentrations." *Cancer Epidemiology, Biomarkers & Prevention.*

Hoyt, Garrett, Matthew S. Hickey, and Loren Cordain. 2007. "Dissociation of the glycaemic and insulinaemic responses to whole and skimmed milk." *British Journal of Nutrition* 175-177.

Jakicic, PhD, John M., PhD, Kelliann K. Davis, PhD, Renee J. Rogers, PhD, Wendy C. King, PhD, Marsha D. Marcus, PhD, RD, Diane Helsel, PhD, RD, LDN, Amy D. Rickman, PhD, Abdus S. Wahed, and PhD, Steven H. Belle. 2016. "Effect of Wearable Technology Combined With a Lifestyle Intervention on Long-term Weight Loss: The IDEA Randomized Clinical Trial." *JAMA* 1161-1171.

Kearns, DDS, MBA, Cristin E., PhD, MSW, MPH, Laura A. Schmidt, and PhD, Stanton A. Glantz. 2016. "Sugar Industry and Coronary Heart Disease Research." *JAMA Internal Medicine* 1680-1685.

Kott, Anne, and MPA, Deirdre Fruh. 2009. *2009 Almanac of Chronic Disease.* Partnership to Fight Chronic Disease.

Kurek, M., B. Przybilla, K. Hermann, and I. Ring. 1992. "Logo International Archives of Allergy and Immunology." *International Archives of allergy and Immunology* 115–120.

Lichtenstein, PhD, Paul, MD, PhD, Niels V. Holm, MD, PhD, Pia K. Verkasalo, MSc, Anastasia Iliadou, MD, PhD, Jaakko Kaprio, MD, PhD, Markku Koskenvuo, PhD, Eero Pukkala, MSc, Axel Skytthe, and MD, PhD, Kari Hemminki. 2000. "Environmental and Heritable Factors in the Causation of Cancer — Analyses of Cohorts of Twins from Sweden, Denmark, and Finland." *The New England Journal of Medicine* 78-85.

Lilburn, The Fitness Center of. 2016. *Pop Tarts are Healthy, Salmon is Not? The Crazy FDA Guidelines That Need to Be Revamped.* Accessed March 2019. https://tfcoflilburn.com/pop-tarts-are-healthy-salmon-is-not-the-crazy-fda-guidelines-that-need-to-be-revamped/.

Ma, Jing, Edward Giovannucci, Michael Pollak, June M. Chan, Michael J. Gaziano, Walter Willett, and Meir J. Stampfer. 2001. "Milk Intake, Circulating Levels of Insulin-Like Growth Factor-I, and

Risk of Colorectal Cancer in Men." *Jurnal of the National Cancer Institute* 1330–1336.

Medicine, Institute of. 2010. *The Healthcare Imperative: Lowering Costs and improving Outcomes: workshop Series Summary.* Edited by Pierre L Yong, Robert S Saunders and LeighAnne Olsen. Washington, D.C.: The National Academies Press.

Medina, John. 2014. *Brain Rules for Baby (Updated and Expanded): How to Raise a Smart and Happy Child from Zero to Five.* Pear Press.

Millard, Claire, Michael Ferriter, Sarah J. Calver, and Graham G. Connell-Jones. 2008. "Gluten- and casein-free diets for autistic spectrum disorder." *Cochrane database of systematic reviews (Online)*, February. doi:10.1002/14651858.CD003498.pub3.

Nestle, PhD, MPH, Marion. 2006. "Food Marketing and Childhood Obesity — A Matter of Policy." *The New England Journal of Medicint* 2527-2529.

Paronen, J., M. Knip, E. Savilahti, S. M. Virtanen, J. Ilonen, H. K. Akerblom, and O. Vaarala. 2000. "Effect of cow's milk exposure and maternal type 1 diabetes on cellular and humoral immunization to dietary insulin in infants at genetic risk for type 1 diabetes. Finnish Trial to Reduce IDDM in the Genetically at Risk Study Group." *Diabetes* 1657-1665.

Prevention, Centers for Disease Control and. 2016. *Obesity and Overweight.* June 13. Accessed March 2019. https://www.cdc.gov/nchs/fastats/obesity-overweight.htm.

Promotion, National Center for Chronic Disease Prevention and Health. 2019. *Health and Economic Costs of Chronic Diseases.* February 11. Accessed April 2019. https://www.cdc.gov/chronicdisease/about/costs/index.htm.

Ratey, John J. 2013. *Spark: The Revolutionary New Science of Exercise and the Brain.* Little, Brown and Company;.

Schauer, MD, MSc, Daniel P., MD, MPH, David E. Arterburn, MD, Edward H. Livingston, MD, David Fischer, and MD, MS, Mark H. Eckman. 2010. "Decision Modeling to Estimate the Impact of Gastric Bypass Surgery on Life Expectancy for the Treatment of Morbid Obesity." *JAMA Surgery* 57-62.

Schneider, MD, Marcie Beth, and MD, Holly J. Benjamin. 2011. "Sports Drinks and Energy Drinks for Children and Adolescents: Are They Appropriate?" *Pediatrics: Official Journal of the american Academy of Pediatrics.*

Sen, Tanusree, Carolina R. Cawthon, Benjamin Thomas Ihde, Andras Hajnal, Patricia M. DiLorenzo, Claire B. de La Serre, and Krzysztof Czaja. 2017. "Diet-driven microbiota dysbiosis is associated with vagal remodeling and obesity." *Physiology & Behavior* 305-317.

Siddique, Haroon. 2016. "Protein hype: shoppers flushing money down the toilet, say experts." *Guardian News & Media Limited,* December 26.

Sørensen, DrMed, Thorkild I. A., Gert G. Nielsen, LicScient, Per Kragh Andersen, and MA, FilDr, Thomas W. Teasdale. 1988. "Genetic and Environmental Influences on Premature Death in Adult Adoptees." *The New England Journal of Medicine* 727-732.

Statista. 2019. *Prescription drug expenditure in the United States from 1960 to 2019 (in billion U.S. dollars).* Accessed April 2019. https://www.statista.com/statistics/184914/prescription-drug-expenditures-in-the-us-since-1960/.

Stuff, Daily Good. 2018. *The food pyramid, signaling system, hand system and plate model, four are the simplest sense of proper nutrition.* May 4. Accessed March 2019. http://dailygoodstuff.net/the-food-pyramid-signaling-system-hand-system-and-plate-model-four-are-the-simplest-sense-of-proper-nutrition/.

The Washington Post Company. 2004. *Pharma Ethics: Merck CEO Resigns – Vioxx deceptive Marketing / AIDS drug experiments*

Foster Kids. Accessed March 2019. https://ahrp.org/pharma-ethics-merck-ceo-resigns-vioxx-deceptive-marketing-aids-drug-experiments-foster-kids/.

The Wellness Practice Global Self Health Corp. 2013. *Innate Choice: The Essential Nutrient System.* Accessed March 2019. http://www.innatechoice.com/viewarticle.cfm?id=3478C647-1E4F-AFAF-04C5DBDA64374214&return=/omega_plus_d.cfm&ref=&plid=.

Weintraub, Pamela. 2010. "The Doctor Who Drank Infectious Broth, Gave Himself an Ulcer, and Solved a Medical Mystery." *Discover Magazine*, April 8.

World Cancer Research Fund. 2018. *Diet, Nutrition, Physical Activity and Cancer: a Global Perspective: The Third Expert Report.* May. Accessed April 2019. https://www.wcrf.org/dietandcancer.

Zyrowski, Nick. 2017. *How To Beat Fatigue And Recover Like Wolverine.* Accessed March 2019. https://blog.biostrap.com/posts/how-to-beat-fatigue-and-recover-like-wolverine.

About the Author

Dr. Czys is a professional speaker, the founder of Eupraxia, founder of Physics Nutrition, and most importantly, a husband and father of two little angels (monsters). He is obsessed with exposing the lies of mainstream nutrition and exercise advice and providing people with the truth they are looking for. In the rare occasion when both kids are sleeping, you'll find him at his gym, Eupraxia, or outdoors working on his farm.

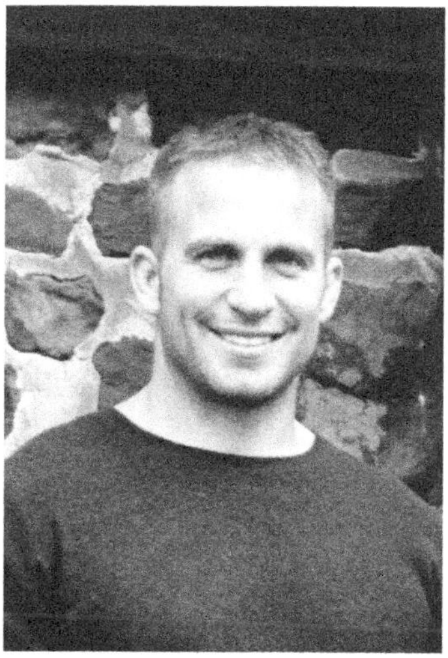

Made in United States
Orlando, FL
08 November 2023

38719503R00139